T5-AFS-403

h

The History of Lithium Therapy

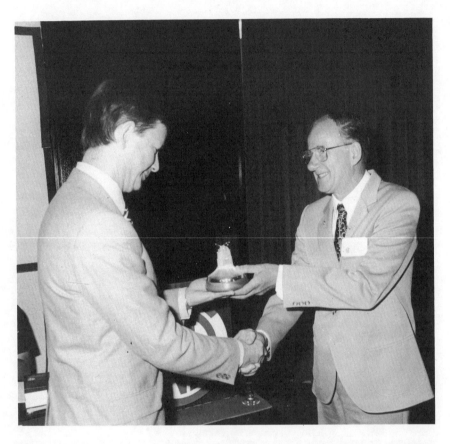

Professor Mogens Schou, today's foremost exponent of lithium therapy, receives the first John Cade Memorial Award from Dr John Cade, son of J. F. J. Cade who first clearly established the antimanic properties of lithium. The award was made at the Congress of the Collegium Internationale Neuro-Psychopharmacologicum in Jerusalem, 1982.

THE HISTORY OF LITHIUM THERAPY

F. Neil Johnson

Department of Psychology
University of Lancaster

MACMILLAN

First published 1984 by
Scientific and Medical Division
THE MACMILLAN PRESS LTD
London and Basingstoke
Companies and representatives throughout the world

Filmsetting by Vantage Photosetting Co Ltd
Eastleigh and London

Printed in Hong Kong

British Library Cataloguing in Publication Data
Johnson, F. Neil
The history of lithium therapy.
1. Lithium—Therapeutic use—History
I. Title
616.89'18   RC483.5.L5
ISBN 0–333–36942–4

My dearest Nete and Mogens

It has been the source of great pleasure to me to write his history, and I can hope for no greater reward than th t it will afford something of the same pleasure to you. It is offered to both of you in the friendship that you ha e so generously and without hesitation given to me.

A man may in his life do many things, own muc , and acquire abilities and expertise in many spheres, but in the end he is to be judged it is not according to h s own achievements that it should be done, but rathe by the friends that are his. Robert Louis Stevenson knew his to be one of the great truths when he asked, 'Of wh t shall a man be proud, if he is not proud of his friends?'

This history is to me a matter of pride – no because I have written it, but because I have two such friends to whom, with this letter, I can most affectionat y dedicate it.

Neil

Contents

Preface

I am not sure exactly when the idea of writing *The History of Lithium Therapy* first occurred to me. I think that it must, perhaps, have been something that grew gradually over the twelve or so years of my association with lithium therapy, although latterly – and particularly since the death in 1980 of John Cade, a man I was both fortunate and proud to count a friend – I have become more and more clearly aware of the personalities behind the clinical and experimental studies which have provided the context for my own work.

Between September 1980 and August 1981 I took sabbatical leave from the University of Lancaster and spent the greater part of that time as a Visiting Research Scientist at the Centre de Recherche Delalande, near Paris. A sabbatical year is traditionally a time for reflection and for taking a longer perspective on one's subject, and somehow, being out of my own country heightened this feeling of wanting to reappraise my work in relation to the general ebb and flow of ideas about lithium. I started to write around to a large number of individuals whom I knew to have been involved at some stage or another in the lithium story, in order to get their views on what had occurred and why, who had said what and to whom, and in general to try to reconstruct the social and personal background to those events which I had encountered in the sterile, impersonal medium of the scientific literature. The response to my letters was patchy: some of those to whom I wrote had, predictably, a lot to say, but others had, less predictably perhaps, little. A few did not reply at all. However, enough came across my desk to convince me that the project of writing a formal history of lithium therapy was not only worthwhile but, more importantly if I was going to give my time to it, a viable proposition; I also felt that there was much that could be added to the few outline accounts that had already appeared, from time to time, in the literature.

I received encouragement in all this from a number of directions. The Lithium Corporation of America made me a modest, but extremely useful, award of travel funds to allow me to visit one or two figures of major historical importance to discuss their roles in the development of lithium therapy and to have access to their correspondence files: I am pleased to be able to take this opportunity of thanking Mr Harold Andrews, the Corporation's President, for his generosity in making this support available and for the keen personal interest that he has shown in the *History*.

Dr Amdi Amdisen, of Aarhus University Institute of Psychiatry, upon learning of my plans immediately threw his energies behind the project and, with an enthusiasm which quite amazed me, gathered a huge quantity of material on the pre-Cade phase of the history of lithium. He coined the term 'the first era of lithium in medicine' to describe this period, and I have adopted this as the title to Chapter 2 which owes so much to his efforts. Indeed, it was not only factual information that Amdi provided; he was a constant source of ideas and suggestions and a most critical and exacting reader of the various drafts through which Chapter 2 went. I have seldom enjoyed a collaboration so much and I acknowledge it here with great pleasure.

When the first draft of the *History* was completed, I sent copies of the relevant pages to all those whose names were mentioned, with a request for comments, corrections, additions, and so on. In this way, I hope that I have managed to keep the record as accurate as possible. Many of those contacted replied with new material which was then incorporated into the text, and I greatly appreciate this enrichment of my writing.

Of course, any historical account is bound to possess a considerable element of interpretation if it is to have any sense of continuity and narrative style rather than being merely a set of facts loosely bound together with limp linguistic threads, and this may involve its own hazards. I hope, however. that I have been as objective as possible in setting down the record, but I readily recognise that there will be some who will feel that I have done less than justice to this or that part of the story, or that distortions have occurred in the way I have emphasised other aspects. I can offer in mitigation only that such errors, if errors they be, were committed in good faith, and add that I am not by nature an historian, this being my first – and maybe my only – excursion into that field of activity.

I have placed the greatest emphasis in the *History* on the earliest days of lithium therapy, making only brief mention of developments and trends that occurred in the period after the establishment of lithium as a prophylactic agent against recurrent depression. I make no apology for this. As editor of three texts on modern lithium therapy and the organiser of the First British Lithium Congress some years ago, I feel that I have done my bit as far as the present is concerned and in the *History* I make my offering to the past, leaving the present, for once, to take care of itself.

If the *History* should prove to be of any value to the student of the history of medicine, or of the history of science more broadly conceived, I shall be pleased. Those who see science and its metamorphoses as reflections of general trends in social history, have a breadth of vision that I envy but cannot emulate: I state the lithium story as I see it, and I leave it to these gifted others to draw the social lessons. My own intention is much more modest. I have set about my task with the simple aim of entertaining and of telling a story that I find quite fascinating. I am, however, hardly unbiased in my view of the importance of lithium – the 'king of drugs' as my good friend Gianpaolo Minnai calls it – and I can only guess at the interest which all this may hold for others.

I must add a brief word about the dedication of this book to Nete and Mogens Schou. I have known Mogens now for a number of years and have not only found stimulation in his great scientific integrity but warmth in the sincerity of his friendship which he so generously offered. Mogens, as everyone who knows *anything* about lithium surely knows, has been the driving force behind the modern use of lithium on a worldwide scale. It is a fact which hardly needs repeating, but I repeat it now and will again, because he has been responsible, more than any other single individual, for bringing about what Ronald Fieve has called the 'third revolution in psychiatry'; I forget what the first two were, but no one, and least of all the many thousands of patients who have benefited from lithium treatment, could – or should – forget the third, or the man behind it.

Oh, of course Mogens was not alone. Of course his message has been based just as much on the work of others as upon his own studies – as he is the first and most insistent in acknowledging; but always it was he who had the vision and the gift of seeing the glint of gold amongst the pebbles in the stream. And behind the man, his wife: what can I say of Nete? A gracious and charming lady, she combines gentleness of manner with a quiet inner strength; indefatigable in her own independent work in bringing practical help to the parents of handicapped children in Denmark, she is fiercely loyal to her husband and his mission. It was natural that I should wish to dedicate this book to Nete and Mogens, for without them lithium might never have progressed beyond being a minor medical curiosity, briefly intriguing but soon forgotten: the history of a stillborn idea would have been a sorry thing indeed.

To all those friends and colleagues who have made substantial contributions to the *History* I express my deepest gratitude; to those who, unbidden, wrote to me to offer their reminiscences and many documents of historical interest, I also extend my thanks. All these willing collaborators are too many to mention individually and I hope that they will forgive me for not doing so – it in no way diminishes my debt to them.

My Editorial Assistant, Julie West, again made a vital contribution to the work: her quiet efficiency is something which I often take for granted but which I could not function without. Delandale Laboratories, makers of Priadel, kindly provided the funding for editorial assistance and so once more have assisted in the dissemination of knowledge about lithium. The typing was done by Anne Parker and Margaret Gill whose skills in handling a capricious word processor restored my confidence in the belief that maybe the machines have not yet taken over the world. They never once complained about the state of my handwritten copy, or my demands for constant revisions of the manuscript, though they had every right to do so, and their typing was, as always, quick and accurate.

My main support throughout this task has, however, come from my wife Susan and my children Jenny and Reuben; I need hardly say, though I do, that no matter what other inducements there might have been to write this book, without *their* encouragement it could not, and would not, have been done.

Historian I may not be, but history I find a graceful and refined pursuit; to relax and to take stock; to review and to reflect; to contemplate and to reconstruct – these are intellectual pleasures of a rare kind. I have heard it said, however, that such things are mere scholarly diversions, more suited to an earlier and gentler age: the future calls us to make haste and there is no time to look back. I would like to think that this is not entirely true and that out of the study of history may emerge not only a better understanding of our present situation but a clearer view of the path ahead.

Lancaster, 1983   F.N.J.

Prologue

In the United Kingdom of Great Britain and Northern Ireland, one person in about two thousand is regularly taking tablets containing a salt of the metallic element, lithium. The figure is likely to be much the same in the USA, Canada, Germany, Australia, and a number of other civilised nations, and may be even higher in certain countries, such as Denmark.

For thirty thousand people in the UK alone to be receiving treatment with lithium salts, the reason has to be a good one – and it is. These chemical substances, though deceptively simple in their constitution when compared with other drugs, provide effective control of one of the most crippling of psychiatric disturbances.

Lithium salts are prescribed, in the great majority of cases, for the treatment of what is commonly called *manic–depression* or more accurately *recurrent endogenous affective disorder*. This condition is characterised by periodic bouts of depressed or elevated mood, and may be either unipolar (periods of disturbed mood – depression or mania – alternating with periods of apparent normality) or bipolar (depression and mania alternating with each other, with periods of apparent normality also occurring). So successful have lithium salts been in the control of these distressing psychiatric conditions, that they are now widely regarded as providing the treatment of choice for patients who could otherwise look forward only to a life dominated by uncertainty about their mental stability and by the likelihood – certainty even – of periodic confinements in hospital.

At the present time, lithium salts rank amongst the most highly regarded of the pharmaceutical agents available to the modern psychiatrist in his battle against mental illness, but, as in so many success stories, the path to the top has not always been a smooth, nor particularly direct, one.

The story of the introduction of lithium into psychiatry is a fascinating one, providing insights not only into the way in which new ideas originate and develop in biomedical science, but also into the social and historical forces which help to shape those ideas and to determine their general acceptability.

The impact of lithium therapy on contemporary psychiatry

Modern psychiatric practice depends heavily upon a wide range of phar-macological products – tranquillisers, sedatives, antidepressants, anticon-vulsants, and so on; indeed, so essential are these agents to effective treatment that their use has become assimilated into the whole theoretical basis of psychopathology, and the responsiveness, or otherwise, of a condi-tion to a particular drug is now an important element in differential diagnosis. We are, however, apt to forget that this situation has existed for only thirty years or so, and that before 1950 drug therapy was the exception rather than the rule in psychiatric institutions: custodial care, physical restraint, and the isolation of patients from their normal environment, were the main, and sometimes the only, tools available to the clinician.

The salts of lithium, introduced into modern psychiatric treatment in 1949, were in the forefront of the psychotherapeutic revolution (the phenothiazines were not introduced until some four years later) and whilst the early years of their use were bedevilled by a series of unfortunate cases of toxicity and even the occasional fatality, the refinement of techniques for monitoring serum lithium levels and for assessing the onset of intoxication has resulted in lithium being one of the most widely used of all present day psychoactive agents.

In assessing the impact which drugs have made upon the practice and theory of psychiatry, lithium provides probably the most interesting and cogent case study.

The early part of the twentieth century saw psychiatry dominated by the ideas of Freud and his followers. The more empirically-based findings of academic psychology made little headway against the shrewd clinical in-sights which Freud brought to his writings, and although Freud himself constantly acknowledged the origins of his ideas in neurology and Darwi-nian evolutionary theory, the imagination of public and psychiatrists alike was captured by those elements of his model of the psyche which least reflected their biological foundations.

All this was changed with the advent of drug treatment. The demonstra-tion that mania was diminished in intensity and in episodic duration follow-ing the administration of lithium salts, and that recurrent periods of depres-sion were, by the same treatment, eliminated prophylactically, could neither be lightly dismissed nor easily reconciled with psychoanalytic notions of the nature of affect. If affective disorders could be eliminated by the simple expedient of administering a chemical substance, did this not suggest that the basis of these disorders might take a chemical form? And not only that; might affect, mood, emotion, and the whole gamut of human conscious experience, be translated into chemical terms? At a stroke, the elusive, aetherial Freudian psyche was replaced as the primary object of attention in psychiatry by the polyphasic, physico-chemical system called the brain. Psychiatry came of age, and took its place amongst the biological sciences.

The idea that psychopathological states are correlated with, and possibly caused by, chemical events, could as easily have come from studies of chlorpromazine, reserpine, amphetamine, or any other drug, as from work on lithium, but lithium has a characteristic possessed by none of these other agents – simplicity of chemical structure. Whereas most psychoactive drugs have molecular structures of often considerable complexity, lithium is an element and hence of the simplest possible molecular form. Not only that, but lithium is closely related to the alkali metals, sodium and potassium, both of which are well known to have virtually ubiquitous presence in biological tissues and fluids.

In the early years of lithium research it was felt that the psychiatrically useful effects of lithium might be related to a simple replacement of sodium or potassium, or both, by lithium. If this were so, then the physiological basis of affect might be identified with a specificity which, before the advent of lithium therapy, had not been thought possible. The fact that we now know this to have been misplaced optimism (the physiological and biochemical consequences of lithium action being no less varied and complex than those of any other drug used in psychiatric treatment) in no way diminishes the importance of the enthusiasm which was thereby engendered.

Lithium became the focus of attention of research workers from a wide array of disciplines. Pharmacologists, biochemists, physiologists, psychiatrists, psychologists, and many others, joined forces in the search of the century – the search for the key to mental illness.

Many bridges were built between the different disciplines of the biological sciences as a result of a common interest of research workers in the problem of lithium. From 1949 onwards, the annual number of publications dealing with aspects of the biology of lithium increased exponentially in a manner little short of dramatic.

It was probably the advent of lithium therapy which, like no other single event, led to psychiatry becoming truly interdisciplinary, a trend which, once started, spread to all aspects of psychiatric practice and theory, with far-reaching consequences.

It is typical of any new and effective drug therapy that once it has become established in the treatment of one disease there is a move to test its usefulness in a variety of different conditions. This is exemplified in a very clear way by what has happened to lithium.

Whilst the major indication for lithium is in the treatment of recurrent endogenous affective disorders, it has nevertheless been used, with varying degrees of success, in other psychiatric and non-psychiatric conditions. Two things stem from this. In the first place, the fact that two symptomatically different disease entities respond to the same treatment suggests that they may possess some commonality of mechanism; if the mechanism underlying one disease is known, it therefore follows that some clue is gained about the mechanism underlying the other. Secondly, the identification of processes which appear in two, three, or even more, otherwise separate and distinct conditions, suggests a new basis for a classification of psychopathological states on other than exclusively symptomatic criteria, and there follows pressure to move from a psychiatric taxonomy of a purely descriptive nature to one based upon dysfunction and emphasising mechanism.

Clinical research with lithium has added, and continues to add, to our knowledge about the kinds of processes which, when disturbed, give rise to mental illness; the information so gained has implicated physiological and biochemical systems (thyroid function, cyclic adenosine monophosphate, mechanisms of circadian and other forms of periodicity, magnesium-dependent enzymes, central processing of information, and so on) which were hitherto either not suspected as having any connection with psychopathology, or were suspected only upon slender evidence.

There can be no doubt that research on all aspects of the affective disorders has been greatly stimulated by the demonstration of the effectiveness of lithium in the treatment of these conditions. The intensification of research effort goes far beyond the mere establishment, by clinical trials, that lithium is indeed effective.

Work with lithium has demonstrated, with a greater degree of clarity than has been shown by any other form of treatment, that mania and depression are closely linked conditions and, in all probability, share a common underlying mechanism. The question of how one mechanism can manifest itself in such different sets of symptoms, and the associated question of what kind of process is involved in switching from one form of overt expression to the other, are of fundamental inportance, and work with lithium provides a useful tool in the search for the answers.

The intense interest generated by lithium therapy has led to several surveys, in the form of detailed review articles and edited texts, which have attempted to impose some superordinate structure on to the subject and to provide a taxonomy or framework against which future work and findings may be assessed.

Because lithium is, if wrongly or carelessly used, such a poisonous element, the issues of absolute and relative contra-indications, side effects, incipient and actual intoxication, and techniques for monitoring the patient's progress, have figured prominently in all taxonomies of the practicalities of lithium treatment.

Lithium therapy can be taken as a model in discussions of pharmacotherapy in psychiatric practice: it embodies – often in a very clear way – all the problems and issues which arise in drug treatment. There can be no doubt that the attention paid to lithium has made psychiatrists more aware of the many considerations which have to be taken into account in the prescription and administration of drug therapies.

Depression is a crippling condition. It results not only in the annual loss of many millions of man-hours in industry, but also in the dislocation of family units, with all the attendant costs upon the social services which such disruption entails. Recurrent conditions which, like recurrent endogenous depression, require constant rehospitalisation, make demands upon hospital facilities here and now and also pre-empt those same facilities for an indeterminate number of future occasions, thereby limiting the amount of forward planning which is possible by health authorities.

Lithium therapy is not only relatively cheap, both in terms of the basic cost of its raw materials and as regards the personal and hospital facilities required for its administration, it also removes the burden of recurrent costs by acting prophylactically against conditions which, without such treatment, would demand repeated hospital admission.

It is certain that in countries where the systems of health care in general, and psychiatric services in particular, are stretched to breaking point, the introduction of lithium therapy has led to a significant lessening of demands made upon scarce resources and to the possibility of at least modest expansion in other forms of treatment which might otherwise not have been feasible.

Lithium therapy has made a significant contribution to modern psychiatry, both in relation to its specific uses in alleviating recurrent endogenous affective disorders, and in stimulating psychiatric research and practice more generally. The full extent of that contribution may never be accurately evaluated but there can be no doubt that without the discovery of the therapeutic effectiveness of lithium salts the development of psychiatric treatment would have been far less extensive than has actually been the case.

The history of lithium therapy

The outlines of the history of lithium therapy have been briefly sketched on a number of occasions, and what might be called the 'official' version is now familiar to almost everyone who prescribes or carries out research on lithium; and to be sure, in certain details it is accurate enough. However, no cursory account can hope to capture the full complexity of what actually happened, or to trace the more elusive lines of influence which, on closer inspection, appear like threads of a spiderweb, linking idea with idea, and investigator with investigator.

This, then, is the full story – or at least, as full as it has been possible to make it, because historically important records and documents are only with hindsight recognised as such and tend to become lost or destroyed *en route* to achieving that status; and human memory is a frail and fickle thing (not to say selective) which often represents what, in a more accommodating world, *would* have happened, rather than what, in this imperfect world, actually did.

1

The discovery of lithium

The new minerals

Off the eastern coast of Sweden in the immediate vicinity of Stockholm there are numerous islands, for the most part rocky and rich in certain minerals. On the island of Utö, iron ore was mined during the eighteenth and nineteenth centuries, and it was in the waste material excavated from the iron mines that the ores containing the element lithium were first found. Their discoverer was Joze Bonifacio de Andrada e Silva,[1] a Brazilian scientist undertaking a geological and mineralogical expedition to a number of European countries under the auspices of the Portuguese Academy of Sciences.

De Andrada named two new minerals found on Utö and certain other Swedish islands; one he called 'petalite' and the other 'spodumene'. The first account of these substances appeared in 1800[2] when a letter from de Andrada to a German mine surveyor was published in a German journal.

The discovery was not, however, followed up, and for seventeen years little more was heard about petalite so that its actual existence became a matter for some doubt. In 1817 petalite was again found on Utö, this time by a Swede, E. T. Svedenstjerna,[3] who immediately sent samples to various acquaintances in Sweden and in other countries.

Analysis of petalite and the discovery of lithium

One of the eventual recipients of a piece of petalite was the Reverend Edward Clarke[4] who received it from Dr Ingle, a colleague in the University of Cambridge. Clarke immediately published a description[5] of the mineral, and of an analysis which he had performed of its constituents. According to his calculations, petalite consisted of silica (80 per cent), alumina (15 per cent), manganese (2.5 per cent), and water (0.75 per cent), but a small proportion (1.75 per cent) remained unaccounted for and unidentified. Clarke did not concern himself much with this small but puzzling residuum, possibly because one of his colleagues, referred to simply as Mr Holme, noticed no such loss in the analysis, reporting only the presence of silica, alumina, manganese and water.

Clarke concluded that whilst the mineral which he had described had indeed been received from Sweden under the name of petalite, it might not actually be the same as the substance described by de Andrada[6] and he added:

> Should this prove to be true, as it will be necessary to bestow some name upon it, we are desirous of calling it *Berzelite*, in honour of the illustrious chemist who presides over the analytical researches of the country in which it was discovered.[7]

The mineral was indeed petalite, but Clarke's reference to Berzelius turned out to be curiously prophetic.

In France, at about the same time, Nicolas-Louis Vauquelin[8] had also come into possession of one of Svedenstjerna's samples of petalite. Ten grammes of the mineral were given to Vauquelin by a colleague, M. Gillet-Laumont who had received it directly from Svedenstjerna. Like Clarke, Vauquelin analysed the sample, finding silica (78 per cent), alumina (13 per cent), some iron oxide and chalk, and an unexplained residual portion of as much as 7 per cent.[9]

By means of subsequent analyses, Vauquelin came to the conclusion that the unknown portion of petalite consisted of an alkaline substance, but the quantity was too small for him to determine its precise chemical nature. He thought it might be potassium: 'J'écrivis à M. Gillet-Laumont que je croyais que la pétalite contenait de la potasse'.[10]

Meanwhile, in Sweden, the problem had already been solved. A young chemist by the name of Johan August Arfwedson,[11] working in the laboratory of Berzelius,[12] had bent his considerable analytical skills to determining the constitution of petalite.[13]

After fusing the petalite with potassium carbonate, Arfwedson estimated the silica content and then took out the alumina by precipitation with ammonium carbonate. The silica and alumina together accounted for 96 per cent of the total sample, leaving an unusually large proportion, 4 per cent, as unidentified 'loss'. Arfwedson then varied the procedure, first of all using barium carbonate to decompose the petalite and then adding sulphuric acid in excess to remove the silica, alumina and barium sulphate. The solution was reduced by evaporation and heated to drive off the ammonium salts. A white residue remained. Soluble in water, this powder failed to respond to the usual tests for either potassium or magnesium (precipitation with excess tartaric acid or platinum chloride, respectively), and was therefore presumed to be sodium sulphate. However, if this had been correct, Arfwedson's total analysis for petalite would have been in the region of 105 per cent. Thinking that an error must have occurred somewhere in the analytic procedure, Arfwedson repeated the analysis on two further occasions, but each time he was forced to the same conclusion: in addition to alumina and silica, petalite contained something else, and whatever it was, it was not potassium, magnesium or sodium.

Reporting these findings for the first time in the *Afhandling i Fysik, Kemi och Mineralogi*[14] in 1818,[15] Arfwedson proposed that a new alkali had been discovered and recorded that Berzelius had suggested for it the name 'lithion' after the Greek word for stone, to signify its mineral origins.

The news of Arfwedson's discovery became known to Vauquelin in advance of its appearance in print, and Vauquelin recorded the fact in his paper of 1817.[16] He noted that after he had written to Monsieur Gillet-Laumont (who had provided the petalite) to say that the unexplained portion of petalite was probably a potassium salt, Arfwedson's conclusions reached him:

Quelques jours après, M. Gillet-Laumont recut de M. Sudenstierna, son correspondant en Suède, la nouvelle que M. Arfredon avait trouvé dans la pétalite un alcali nouveau auquel M. Berzelius avait donné le nom de *lithion*, parce qu'il a été trouvé dans le règne minéral.[17]

Edward Clarke, on receiving the news from Svedenstjerna, hastened to publish the information in English,[18] adding that he felt that Arfwedson had missed the manganese content of petalite. In fact, Clarke was quite wrong in this. His repeated suggestion that the mineral ore be named Berzelite 'because it is evident that the old name of *petalite* was not applied to the mineral containing *lithion*',[19] failed to be adopted.

Berzelius himself was not too happy with the name 'lithion' for the new alkali, remarking[20] that the termination of the word was peculiarly Swedish and might require some modification to fit easily into other languages. 'Lithine' was suggested for French and 'lithina' for English, the latter being adopted by Thomas Thompson in his review of scientific achievements in 1817,[21] but only for the alkali salt and not for the metal 'to which the name of *lithium* will of course be given'.[22] There is often some confusion as to exactly what Berzelius was intending to name when he proposed the term 'lithion'. In fact, this was meant to apply to the alkali found by Arfwedson and not to the metallic principle which had not, at that stage, been isolated.[23]

The analyses of petalite were subsequently repeated by other investigators. The distinguished German chemist C. G. Gmelin of Tübingen, provided a very detailed account[24] in which he explained the finding by Clarke[25] of a proportion of manganese in petalite, as arising from the use of an impure sample of the mineral. Gmelin went on to give an extensive account of the properties of a large number of lithium salts.

The discovery of lithium might, in fact, have occurred somewhat earlier than it did, had a chance observation not been overlooked. Johann Nepomuk von Fuchs,[26] in the course of investigating the colours imparted by various substances to the blowpipe flame,[27] noted that spodumene produced a flame of characteristic reddish hue. Franz von Kobell, the biographer of Fuchs, wrote[28] of this work: 'I remember his expression of chagrin that he had omitted to investigate the cause of this coloration, for he was convinced that otherwise the discovery of lithia would not have escaped him'.[29]

The preparation of lithium metal

Arfwedson himself apparently attempted to isolate lithium metal,[30] but was unsuccessful. However, Sir Humphry Davy, to whom some samples of the newly-discovered lithium salt had been given,[31] prepared a very small quantity of lithium by means of his electrolytic procedure.[32] Lithium carbonate, fused in a small platinum vessel, had an electric current passed through it; the carbonate decomposed with a good deal of flashing and crackling, and the shiny metal remained as a few tiny globules. Within seconds the metal burned in the air and was lost, but for that brief fraction of time the thing was done and Sir Humphry Davy became the first person to see the new element, lightest of all the metals.[33]

A few years later, W. T. Brande,[34] also using an electrolytic process, repeated the separation of lithium using lithium oxide (lithia).

> When lithia is submitted to the action of the Voltaic pile, it is decomposed with the same phenomena as potassa and soda; a brilliant white and highly combustible metallic substance is separated, which may be called *lithium*, the term *lithia* being applied to its oxide.[35]

Again, however, the amount of lithium produced was very small.

It was not until 1855 that Robert Bunsen in collaboration with A. Matthiessen[36] succeeded in producing any appreciable quantity of lithium, which they preserved by placing the freshly-prepared globules of molten metal under petroleum to prevent the otherwise rapid combustion which would take place if the metal were left exposed to the air. This opened the way to a thorough exploration of the properties of lithium metal and its compounds.

Johan August Arfwedson did not, however, live to see the coming of age of his discovery. In 1841 he received the gold medal of the Swedish Academy of Sciences for his services to chemistry in general and his discovery of lithium in particular; he died the same year.

2

The first era in medicine

The work of Alexander Ure

One of the most interesting chapters in the history of medicine opened in 1843 with the presentation to the Pharmaceutical Society of a talk entitled 'Observations and researches upon a new solvent for stone in the bladder', the text of which was subsequently recorded in the *Pharmaceutical Journal and Transactions*.[1] Mr Alexander Ure, surgeon to the Western Ophthalmic Institution, explained how he had come to the conclusion that carbonate of lithia, 'a substance of which no therapeutic application has been heretofore made',[2] could be used to dissolve human urinary calculi. He noted the 'remarkable affinity'[3] of lithium carbonate for uric acid, as demonstrated by the work, some two years earlier,[4] of Dr A. Lipowitz who had found that by boiling crushed lepidolite with uric acid in water lithium urate was formed in solution. Ure then displayed to the members of the Pharmaceutical Society a urinary calculus which had lost five grains in weight after five hours' immersion in a solution of lithium carbonate, and he proposed that injection of lithium carbonate into the urinary bladder might be an effective means of reducing the size of urinary calculi, many of which had high uric acid content. Nothing, he declared, had hindered him from employing such a technique, but the great scarcity of the chemical.[5]

The Chairman of the Pharmaceutical Society, in thanking Mr Ure for his presentation, commented upon the potential importance of the subject, and said that he 'had no doubt that the carbonate of lithium might be obtained without much difficulty if a demand should arise for it'.[6]

In fact, it took several years for the supply to become sufficiently abundant to allow Ure to put his method to the test. In the *Lancet* of 25 August 1860, a report appeared of Ure's litholysis technique[7] which he had commenced to put into practice on 30 May 1859. After emptying the patient's bladder by catheterisation and washing it out with distilled water, a solution of lithium carbonate was introduced. The procedure was repeated on 2 June and thereafter every second or third day over a period of several weeks. The urinary calculus refused, however, to reduce in size. Ure therefore resorted to crushing the stone, using a lithotrite, on a number of occasions. He was not discouraged from his view that the lithium salt had a dissolving action on urinary calculi; it seemed, he said, as though the treatment with lithium carbonate 'had in some measure lessened the cohesion of the concretion, and increased its friability'.[8] Despite this, the patient 'got into a state of extreme depression'[9] and eventually died. The cause of death was not recorded.

Ure injected the lithium carbonate solution directly into the bladder because he felt that oral administration would lead to the formation of an insoluble 'double salt of phosphate of soda and lithia'.[10]

One may ask why it was that lithium carbonate suddenly became available in sufficient quantities for Ure to try out his idea. The *Lancet* provided the answer, noting that the substance had become more abundant 'since the publication of Dr Garrod's work on "Gout"'.[11]

Sir Alfred Garrod and the treatment of gout

When, in 1859, Sir Alfred Baring Garrod wrote his celebrated treatise on the nature, causes and cures of gout,[12] he was undoubtedly aware of, and strongly influenced by, the work of Alexander Ure, particularly since Ure had, in 1844–45, made quite explicit an association between uric acid accumulation and gout.[13]

Garrod repeated the experiments of Ure, but on phalanges from gouty patients rather than on bladder stones.

> To show the power which carbonate of lithia possesses in rendering urate of soda soluble, I made the following experiment: A metacarpal bone was selected, having the phalangeal extremity completely infiltrated with gouty deposit; this was placed in a small quantity of cold water, and a few grains of carbonate of lithia added; in the course of two or three days, when the head of the bone was examined, no deposit could be seen, and the cartilage appeared to have been restored to its normal state.[14]

He then went on to develop the view that gout was caused by an accumulation of uric acid in the body and also that this excess uric acid was the cause of certain other symptoms which could be grouped together under the general heading of the *uric acid diathesis*. As he put it, 'the salts of this alkali may prove most powerful in the treatment of gout, and likewise in other affections, the pathology of which is closely connected with an excess of uric acid in the system'.[15]

Garrod was not, by a long way, the first to implicate some kind of chemical concretion around the joints in the aetiology of gout; such a notion had found expression in the eighteenth century and was, indeed, fully accepted in the writings of Dr William Cullen, author of several influential textbooks published between 1773 and 1780.[16] Garrod's contribution, however, took the idea further.

Because uric acid was soluble to only a slight degree, Garrod suggested that its elimination from the body might best be achieved by converting it to the form of a soluble salt and, following Ure's suggestion, proposed that the lithium salt would be the most appropriate in this respect. Garrod's tabulation of uric acid salts and their relative solubilities in distilled water, presented in 1883,[17] showed lithium urate to be just over twice as soluble as its nearest rival, the potassium salt, and thirty-six times as soluble as uric acid itself. Garrod therefore recommended the use of orally administered lithium salts, despite Ure's feeling that the oral route would be an ineffective way of introducing lithium into the body because of the formation of insoluble salts with body phosphates.

Antecedents of Garrod's ideas

It is generally regarded as established that Garrod was the first to give oral lithium therapeutically. In the second edition of his book on gout, Garrod had claimed that, 'the lithia salts can scarcely be said to have been employed therapeutically until recently[18] introduced by myself in the treatment of uric acid gravel and chronic gouty conditions of the habit'.[19] It is, however, possible that some physicians at an even earlier date may have considered the value of giving lithium salts orally, since in a brief report[20] on carbonate of lithia, which appeared in 1860, reference was made to the fact that whilst nothing was known about the internal employment of lithium carbonate at the time that Ure was doing his work, 'Dr Pereira conjectured that by its use the urine would become alkaline, and Aschenbrenner believed that it might be given in from five to ten grains daily'.[21] It is therefore possible that either Pereira or Aschenbrenner (or both) may actually have regarded lithium carbonate as having some kind of medicinal properties, even if they themselves never actually administered it.

Dr Jonathon Pereira was a well-known physician in the first half of the nineteenth century, and co-author of *Elements of Materia Medica and Therapeutics*.[22] In this work he discussed the therapeutic value of saline waters (*aquae salinae*), one group of which comprised the alkaline waters (containing sodium carbonate or bicarbonate as the main ingredient). Of these waters, Pereira wrote that, 'when taken internally, they act on the urinary organs' and he added that, 'they may be employed in calculous complaints connected with lithic acid[23] diathesis, in gout, in dyspesia &c.'[24] It is clear from this that the uric acid diathesis was a concept in current medical usage at least twenty years before Garrod was to expound it in detail (so well known an idea, in fact, that Pereira did not trouble to explain it further to his readers); moreover, the association of gout with the uric acid diathesis undoubtedly predated Garrod's work by at least the same length of time. There is, however, no clear evidence that Pereira ever employed lithium salts therapeutically.[25]

Probably the first formal introduction of alkaline substances into the literature as prophylactic agents in the control of gout was by Dr William Cullen who asserted, in his *First Lines of the Practice of Physic*,[26] published in 1777, that alkalis were apparently efficacious in preventing the return of gouty concretions. Of course, salts of lithium were unknown, as such, in the eighteenth century and so Cullen could make no specific reference to them. Nevertheless, it is clearly of considerable relevance to an understanding of Garrod's work and ideas that similar notions were being aired some sixty or more years earlier.

Whatever the truth of the matter, however, it was Garrod's use of orally administered lithium carbonate in the context of the treatment of gout, which received the greatest public acknowledgement, and although he may not himself have been the originator of the uric acid diathesis concept he was undoubtedly the most eloquent exponent and promulgator of the idea. As a result, knowledge of his work and ideas spread rapidly and widely, as indeed did the use of lithium salts. By the time that his book on gout reached its second edition, only four years after the first,[27] Garrod was able to write:

> These observations led me to propose, in the first edition of the present work, the salts of lithia as valuable remedial agents, and, although I was assured by those most competent to give an opinion on the subject, that it would be almost impossible to procure a single pound of the carbonate of lithia in Europe, I believe I am not in error in stating that notwithstanding its high price, more than a hundred pounds have already been therapeutically employed in this country.[28]

Scope of the uric acid diathesis concept

Garrod's treatise appeared in several editions over a number of years, each being translated into several languages. A French edition appeared in 1867. In 1873, Garrod presented a series of three articles[29] in the *Medical Times and Gazette*, devoted to the subject of the value of lithium salts in the treatment of renal calculus, gravel and gouty deposits, in which articles he again took credit for having introduced lithium salts to the notice of the medical profession. In these extremely interesting accounts of his ideas, Garrod referred to the alkaline properties of lithium salts but commented that as antacid remedies they offered no special advantages. He also noted lithium salts as having marked diuretic properties[30] and proposed that this might be useful in cases in which an alkaline diuretic was indicated. The capacity of lithium salts[31] to render soluble both uric acid and the less soluble urates was, however, seen as their most important feature.

The core of Garrod's argument was neatly summed up in one sentence:

> As the inconveniences which uric acid or its salts cause in the system depend on their very sparing solubility, leading to the formation of calculi, gravel, or gouty deposits, it can be readily understood that an agent possessing the powers of lithium would be likely to prove of considerable advantage in many diseases in which uric acid plays an important part.[32]

The assertion that not only gout but various other conditions would prove amenable to lithium treatment is a very clear indication that the uric acid diathesis concept itself was, in Garrod's view, extendable to a wide range of conditions beyond those of gout and renal calculi, and this notion is crucial in understanding how it eventually came about that lithium was used in the treatment of mental as well as physical conditions. Indeed, in the course of reporting the case histories of a number of patients whom he treated with lithium salts for the alleviation of urinary problems identified as having their origins in uric acid excess, Garrod observed that the cure of the primary symptoms was often also accompanied by improvements in other, less specific ways – including mental changes, such as increased feelings of general well-being.[33]

There can be no doubt that Garrod did indeed envisage the uric acid diathesis as covering a very great variety of diseases, amongst them being disorders of mood; referring to 'gout retroceding to the head'[34] he noted that 'when retrocedent gout attacks the head, apoplexy is commonly induced, but maniacal symptoms occasionally arise';[35] and elsewhere he used the terms 'gouty mania'[36] and 'complete mental derangement'.[37] 'It is', Garrod concluded, 'natural to suppose that gouty patients would from time to time exhibit symptoms other than those of ordinary gout, resulting from the presence of [uric] acid in the system.'[38]

Garrod was certainly acting within a traditional framework when he took the wider view of the uric acid (sometimes called the gouty or rheumatic) diathesis: Copeman[39] writing about the history of gout, noted that the word had its origins in Roman Europe, being derived from *gutta* (meaning 'a drop') in accordance with the idea that one of the four body humours dripped into a joint to cause the swelling and discomfort of gout, and he observed that, 'the implications of this type of pathology were not, however, confined to the joints since such a flow of humours might obviously occur in any part of the body; and so we often meet with references to "gouty" migraine, diarrhoea, haemorrhoids, sciatica, and even gouty paralysis and epilepsy'.[40] Copeman went on to observe that the term 'rheumatism' was also later employed in the context of humoural movements, a point of particular interest in view of the subsequent incorporation of rheumatism within the uric acid diathesis.

In the light of the much later use of lithium as a prophylactic agent against the periodic recurrence of depression, it is worth noting that Garrod himself actually advocated the long-term prophylactic use of lithium salts:

It would naturally be supposed, that lithium salts might prove of advantage in the treatment of both acute and chronic forms of gouty inflammation, and likewise, when administered in the intervals of the attacks, might keep up such a state of the blood as to prevent the recurrence of such inflammatory action.[41]

The proper administration of lithia has a considerable power in preventing the recurrence of gouty paroxysms.[42]

I wish it particularly to be understood, that I do not consider lithia will in any way replace colchicum as a remedy for gouty inflammation; it may prove a valuable adjunct, but its chief use is in chronic gouty cases, to ward off attacks ... it is likewise valuable when administered as part of the prophylactic treatment.[43]

Dissemination of the uric acid diathesis concept

Awareness of the uric acid diathesis concept, as revitalised by Garrod, spread to continental Europe, due mainly to its incorporation into important and influential textbooks such as that first published in 1875 by Arnaldo Cantani, an endocrinologist and Professor and Director of the Naples University Clinic. Cantani's book on the pathology and therapy of metabolic diseases,[44] which was translated from the original Italian into several other languages including German,[45] made extensive and detailed references to Garrod's work and ideas. The physicians of the time were clearly very receptive to such a new, and apparently unifying, concept as the uric acid diathesis, and enthusiastically embraced it, extending it along the lines already foreshadowed in Garrod's and earlier writings to cover a wide variety of symptoms and conditions.

Cantani, whilst himself somewhat critical of the trend for ascribing a wealth of diseases to the rheumatic diathesis, nevertheless gave full documentation of the extensive use of the notion in the 1870s. In particular, in the description of the rheumatic diathesis, several typical depressive symptoms were listed, melancholia being directly mentioned.

Trousseau: manic–depression and the uric acid diathesis

Cantani mentioned briefly the work of Professor A. Trousseau, an influential figure of his time and Head of the Clinic of Medicine of the Hôtel-Dieu,

Paris in the 1860s and 1870s. Trousseau wrote a major medical textbook[46] in which 'folie' and mania were incorporated into the uric acid diathesis; this book was translated into other European languages. Trousseau's description of the uric acid diathesis was fully as detailed and complete as that presented by Garrod. In particular, he recorded both depression and elevated mood as being associated with gout and, by implication, related to the same underlying metabolic cause. It is worth quoting Trousseau extensively on this point:

> parmi les phénomènes prémonitoires de l'attaque de goutte, ce sont les *troubles nerveux* qui sont les plus prononcés. Le goutteux, à cette période du début de son attaque, se plaint de pésanteur de tête, d'inaptitude à toute espèce de travail intellectuel; les modifications dans l'état cérébral se traduisent principalement par une excitabilité nerveuse portée souvent au plus haut degré, aussi bien dans la goutte regulière que dans la goutte irregulière, tout en n'étant jamais plus prononcée que dans cette dernière forme. Cette excitabilité nerveuse se manifeste par les phénomènes les plus variables suivant les individus. C'est un sentiment de malaise indefinissable, d'inquiétude morale; ce sont des changements singuliers survenus dans la caractère. Si, chez quelques-uns on observe une exhaltation de leurs qualités brillantes, il est loin d'en être toujours ainsi. Le plus ordinairement, le goutteux devient morose, d'une susceptibilité, d'une irascibilité qui souvent n'étaient pas dans ces habitudes. C'est tellement là le fait le plus commun, que cette disposition facheuse à la moroscité, à l'irascibilité, est passée comme un proverbe parmi les auteurs qui se sont occupés de la goutte. Cette disposition est parfois tellement exagérée, elle est quelquefois si constante chez certains individus, que, non-seulement ces individus savent par expérience qu'ils vont avoir un accès, parce que depuis quelques jours leur humeur s'aigrit sans raison, mais encore que ceux qui les entourent peuvent prévoir, d'après l'apparition de ces phénomènes moraux, l'imminence de l'attaque, de la même façon que chez quelques femmes la crise cataméniale s'annonce par des changements dans l'état moral.[47]

Of course, if Trousseau believed that mania, even when occurring in isolation from other symptoms, was a manifestation of uric acid imbalance, it is quite possible that he may have attempted to treat it with lithium salts, in which case he would have a good claim to have been the first to use lithium as an acute antimanic agent. Trousseau mentioned 'alkalinization' as an effective treatment for epilepsy, and included developing mania amongst the epileptic equivalents; moreover he recommended morphine as a treatment for rheumatism, and since opium had for some hundred years been used as an antimanic medication[48] it is at least open to conjecture that Trousseau may have transferred the lithium treatment of rheumatism to the treatment of mania, once mania and other mental disturbances had been incorporated into the concept of the rheumatic (uric acid) diathesis.

The writings of John Aulde

A series of three longish articles[49] written by Dr John Aulde of Philadelphia, and published in the *Medical Bulletin* for 1887, provide an unequalled demonstration of the way in which the uric acid diathesis was used at that time as an umbrella concept under which to gather a wide range of complaints. In particular, the presence of mental symptoms indicative of affective disturbance was listed as relatively common: thus, several patients were described as deriving no benefit from their night's rest and as being tired all the time, one as showing 'a marked depression of the vital powers',[50] and still others as having countenances 'bleached and melancholic'[51] or as feeling 'irritable and out of sorts with everybody'.[52] In all cases, treatment with lithium alleviated both physical and mental symptoms rapidly and effectively.

Aulde referred on several occasions to a possible preventative or prophylactic use of lithium bromide, advising certain patients to continue the medication even after apparently being cured. Failure to comply with these instructions led to 'the old trouble coming back',[53] and the need to secure the patient's promise 'to be more docile in future'[54] and to stick to the maintenance treatment regime.

Despite the variability in the symptom patterns, Aulde was prepared to group them all together as exemplifying 'lithaemia, lithiasis, or uric acid diathesis'.[55] He was also open to the suggestion that the most evident symptom in such conditions as rheumatoid arthritis was not necessarily primary in aetiological importance, quoting approvingly a remark made by a Dr Pepper at the First Annual Meeting of the Association of American Physicians, in 1886, to the effect that 'the nervous system may be at the root of, and be the real cause of all these disorders'.[56] At the same meeting a Dr Draper also made a comment which Aulde found worth reporting: 'We have too much limited gout by insisting on the deposit of uric acid in the joints . . . this is, after all, only an epiphenomenon of the disease'.[57]

As an example of the way in which the symptomatology of a patient showing the uric acid diathesis might easily be misdiagnosed, as a result of its relatively nonspecific nature, Aulde reported the case of a female patient who 'during the previous three or four years had consulted no less than six physicians, and according to her statement, every one of them gave her a different disease, while, besides, she had one of her own, which she always kept handy for ordinary occasions'.[58] Lithium bromide, taken for two weeks, successfully eliminated all seven afflictions.

Alexander Haig and the zenith of uric acid

While Sir Alfred Garrod was undoubtedly the prime mover in establishing the title of lithium salts to an important place in medical treatment, major, and arguably comparable, contributions were made by certain other writers in the late nineteenth century. One of these was Alexander Haig, a British physician and author of an influential textbook on the role in illness of uric acid,[59] on which subject he came to be regarded as the primary authority; another was a Danish internist, Carl Lange, who addressed himself primarily to the question of periodic depression as an expression of the uric acid diathesis.

The ideas of Alexander Haig had their origin in a short article which he wrote in the *Practitioner* in 1884,[60] in which he related the occurrence of headache in a male patient to the presence of an 'impurity' in the blood, the source of the impurity lying, in Haig's view, in the patient's diet. Two years later, however, in a follow-up article in the same journal,[61] Haig wrote that he was 'now inclined to believe that it may not be necessary to go beyond our old friend uric acid'.[62] Haig founded this view primarily upon the inclusion of megrim (severe headache) in the uric acid diathesis, along with gout.[63]

In this second article, Haig quoted the view of Dr P. W. Latham[64] that uric acid formation might be prevented by benzoic or salicylic acid or, once formed, destroyed by potassium iodide. This is particularly interesting in view of the introduction into medical treatment of lithium benzoate, salicylate and iodide around this time.[65]

Even more interesting, perhaps, is the fact that Haig clearly bracketed a number of mental problems together with gout and headache and thus, implicitly, regarded them as falling within the ambit of the uric acid diathesis. 'Many symptoms said to be premonitory of gout', he wrote, 'may also precede or accompany the onset of megrim, or gastro-intestinal disturbance, giddiness, irritability, impaired mental vigour, low spirits, restless sleep, unpleasant dreams, numbness, or tingling in the limbs'[66] – all of which added up to quite a neat picture of a depressive reaction.

The first mention which Haig made of lithium occurred in 1888, again in relation to headache and uric acid, in an article in the *Medico-Chirurgical Transactions*.[67] Lithium citrate given orally, he reported, led to a reduced uric acid excretion, a finding which caused him to express some surprise in view of Garrod's demonstration of the extreme solubility of lithium urate and the expectation, therefore, that the administration of lithium salts would lead to increased, not decreased, elimination of uric acid in the form of lithium urate. Haig resolved the problem by concluding that, 'lithia taken internally not only never reaches the uric acid to form a soluble urate, but in forming an insoluble compound with phosphate of soda it practically removes from the blood one of the well-known solvents of uric acid'.[68]

All in all, Haig was decidedly cool towards the likely therapeutic value of lithium:

> With regard to lithia I have very little to say. It was at one time much used,[69] then fell into disuse, and has finally been brought forward again in the treatment of uric acid disease, but there is by no means a unanimous opinion as to its value at the present day.[70]

In a subsequent article[71] in the same year, 1888, Haig explicitly related both depression and manic–depression to uric acid levels in the body. He wrote:

> My researches in the relation of a certain form of headache to the excretion of uric acid showed me among other things that mental depression, and its opposite condition of mental exaltation and sense of well-being, had just as close a relation to the excretion of uric acid, as had headache.[72]

According to Haig, when the blood acidity was raised, the uric acid became less soluble and thus remained in the joints, liver, spleen, and other organs. Alkalinisation of the blood (*except by lithium compounds*) would, on the other hand, be followed by increased solubility of the uric acid and its consequent excretion. High blood levels of uric acid under acid conditions were seen as promoting depression, a lowering of blood uric acid levels being followed by a raising of mood. Patients might therefore be expected to notice an alternation between gouty or rheumatic pains and mental depression.[73] Haig's ideas were developed in a number of articles over the next twelve years, finding their clearest expression in his book *Uric Acid as a Factor in the Causation of Disease* which first appeared in 1892[74] and then in numerous subsequent editions over the next ten or so years.

In all Haig's writings, lithium salts were described as substances diminishing, rather than increasing, the excretion of uric acid. In the fifth edition of *Uric Acid*,[75] Haig noted that:

> lithia . . . relieves arthritis by clearing the blood of uric acid but not as was supposed by eliminating uric acid from the body; we now see that it clears the blood, but retains the uric acid in the body.[76]

By acting to clear the blood, lithium salts should, on Haig's view of the role of uric acid in the causation of depression, act to relieve depressed mood.

> With regard to lithia . . . my results show that it diminishes the excretion of uric acid,[77] and at the same time relaxes the arterioles and quickens the pulse, causes mental well-being and a free flow of urine.[78]

Whilst Haig's views on the role of uric acid in depression were developed gradually over a number of years, and were the result of much careful experimentation, he had actually been preempted in his ideas by Dr Charles Murchison who, in 1874, presented the Croonian Lectures[79] in which he suggested that abnormal breakdown of albuminous material in the liver might lead to an excess of uric acid in the blood (lithaemia). Associated with lithaemia, in Murchison's view, were a variety of mental symptoms including, as primary items, aching limbs and lassitude, headache, sleeplessness, irritability, and depression of spirits. This seems to have been one of the earliest attempts to relate depression to uric acid levels. Nevertheless, it was Haig's detailed and forceful formulation of this idea which was to have the greater impact on medical opinion and research in the late nineteenth and early twentieth centuries.

It is unlikely that Haig was familiar with the work of Dr S. Weir Mitchell, which appeared in the form of a very brief report in 1870 in the *American Journal of the Medical Sciences*.[80] Mitchell reported an anti-epileptic potential of lithium bromide[81] but in several of the case reports which he presented there was some evidence that there may have been a depressive component to the patient's condition: depressive symptoms (sleeplessness, memory impairments, aphasia) and occasionally what may have been depressive equivalents (referred temporal pain, headaches, ringing in the ears) were banished following lithium bromide administration.

Despite his spirited advocacy of uric acid as the causative principle behind many different forms of illness, Haig did not receive universal acclaim for his work. Sir William Roberts was particularly scathing; in a report of a discussion held at the Royal Medical and Chirurgical Society in London early in 1893,[82] it was recorded that:

> Sir William Roberts found that he could scarcely intervene in the discussion with much advantage. He had been following Dr Haig's work for years, but he thought that a too continuous study of one subject led to something like mesmeric dazing and diminished an author's experimental resources.[83]

Sir William added that he felt that uric acid in solution was probably quite harmless and, moreover, he was even 'inclined . . . to believe that if uric acid were withdrawn altogether gout would still remain as a clinical and pathological entity recognisable as such'.[84]

Nevertheless, with the work of Alexander Haig, uric acid reached its highest point in medical theory, and the uric acid diathesis dominated a large area of clinical practice in the nineteenth century; and where the uric acid diathesis was found, lithium was sure to be following.

Carl Lange: the prophylactic treatment of depression

The possible role of the Danish internist Carl Lange in the history of lithium therapy was mentioned by Professor Mogens Schou in 1957[85] when he noted that Lange had published four papers in 1897[86] describing the use of lithium salts in the treatment of conditions involving both gout and mental depression: treatment with lithium, Lange claimed, led to some improvement in depression. The 1897 reports were not, however, the first indications given by Lange of the effectiveness of lithium against depression. Some eleven years earlier, in 1886, he had published a monograph, written in Danish and entitled *Concerning Periodic Depression and its Pathogenesis.*[87] He based his discussion upon observation of a high frequency of masked depressions (non-psychotic slight depression) in his private neurological practice; observing the periodic character of the condition, he also found a substantial increase in urinary sediment which he wrongly believed to be uric acid.[88] The periodicity of the depression, and the urinary sediment, led Lange to incorporate the condition into Garrod's uric acid diathesis and to use prophylactic lithium together with exercise and dietetic measures by way of treatment.

It was in his monograph of 1886[89] that Lange gave the first report of his use of a lithium-containing mixture for the preventive treatment of periodic depression: the mixture included lithium carbonate in quantities which make it highly likely that the therapeutic success which was claimed for it was due almost entirely to the lithium, the patient receiving between 6 and 12 millimoles of lithium daily.[90] The lithium salt was included in accordance with Lange's belief that alkalinisation of the blood would eliminate uric acid and would act prophylactically against recurrence of the clinical symptoms.

The 1886 document is clearly an important one, containing as it does the first unequivocal account of prophylactic drug treatment for an exclusively psychiatric – as distinct from physical – condition, and establishing Carl Lange as one of the most significant forerunners of the modern era of lithium therapy. It is obviously of interest, therefore, to determine what line of influence, if any, may be traced between Lange's work and ideas and the twentieth-century uses of lithium in psychiatric medicine.

Clearly, a pamphlet published in Danish would be likely to have a very restricted audience and hence a limited impact on psychiatric theorising in other countries. However, the 1886 pamphlet was translated into German and published in 1896 in Hamburg and Leipzig[91] where it would certainly have received wide attention.

There can be no doubt that Lange's ideas became quite widely disseminated[92] and were, indeed, very well known to Alexander Haig. In the fifth edition of *Uric Acid,*[93] Haig wrote:

> soon after I wrote my first paper on mental depression[94] ... , Professor Lange, of Copenhagen, kindly wrote to me and sent me a monograph which he published in 1886[95] on periodical depression and its connection with the uric acid diathesis. ... His clinical observations and his treatment of the trouble ran parallel to my own.[96]

Lange, in his turn, later mentioned in a monograph published in 1895[97] 'an English scientist working with uric acid' (presumably Haig).

Lange was also fully aware of the work and ideas of Sir Alfred Garrod, since he gave few details of the mixture containing lithium carbonate, assuming his readers to be thoroughly familiar with its composition as a result of Garrod's writings.

Despite the clear connections between Carl Lange, Alexander Haig and Sir Alfred Garrod, nothing much appears to have been said in the psychiatric literature about Lange's work, and his use of lithium prophylaxis, in particular, seems to have been totally ignored. The final dismissal came in 1938 in an article in the Danish *Ugeskrift for Laeger*,[98] and here there occurs a strange historical coincidence. This article, whilst giving Carl Lange full and glowing credit for the detailed description of endogenous depression which he had presented in the 1886 paper[99], nevertheless did not mention the claims which had been made for the success of the lithium treatment and its success was uncompromisingly denied.[100] The author of the paper was Dr H. I. Schou – father of Professor Mogens Schou, the foremost exponent of modern-day lithium therapy.

Fritz Lange: the acute treatment of depression

Family connections are by no means unknown in the early history of lithium therapy and it is of particular interest in this respect that Carl Lange's brother, (Frederik) Fritz Lange, published in 1894 a book entitled *The Most Important Groups of Insanity*[101] (written in Danish). In it, he described the use of lithium carbonate alone (i.e. not in combination with any other drug) as an acute antidepressant. A good therapeutic response was claimed, this response occurring within a few days of the commencement of treatment.

Like that of his brother, the work of Fritz Lange, after enjoying a brief period of acclaim, was ignored and then eventually forgotten.

Fritz Lange may actually have been pre-dated in his use of lithium as an acute antidepressant, by George Duncan Gibb, a British physician who in 1864 reported to the British Association for the Advancement of Science (the report appearing in print the following year)[102] that lithium bromide 'prepared with the view of treating gout and rheumatism of the throat and neck'[103] had tonic and gentle stimulant properties in small doses. It is possible – though not directly documented – that Gibb made use of these attributes of lithium bromide in treating cases of mild depression: he commented only that it 'may be combined with other agents with advantage',[104] but for what conditions he did not elaborate.

It has already been suggested[105] that Dr Weir Mitchell could have been, in some cases, treating masked depressive components when he used lithium bromide as an anti-epileptic; he was certainly aware that it might have stimulant properties, commenting that he had been struck by the fact that lithium bromide 'seemed to cause a more rapid and intense sleeplessness than the other bromides'.[106]

It cannot, however, be denied that Fritz Lange must be acknowledged as having been the first to make a fully explicit and unequivocal report of a lithium salt used clinically as an acute antidepressant – something which Alexander Haig never did directly.

The unwitting treatment of depression

The erroneous use of lithium salts in the management of various conditions which, in the late nineteenth century, had been assimilated into the uric acid diathesis, may actually have led to the quite accidental treatment – both acute and prophylactic – of depression or manic–depression; in response to a request[107] for ancedotal information about the early uses of lithium, one correspondent gave graphic evidence of this:

> I was born in 1917 and soon afterwards my mother . . . suffered a depressive illness for which she was admitted to [hospital]. . . . When I was quite a young child she suffered from 'gravel' for which she was prescribed lithium citrate and this she took for almost all the rest of her life. . . . Aged 73 she began to be incontinent . . . and at operation [the urologist] removed a pear-sized stone from her bladder. . . . Post-operatively she discontinued the lithium citrate as there seemed no need for it.[108] Six months later . . . she suddenly broke down with agitated depression from which she suffered for seven and a half years until her death.[109]

Mineral springs

Around the time that Garrod, Haig and the Lange brothers were writing it was widely held, both amongst members of the general public and by a considerable number of medical practitioners, that considerable therapeutic benefit was to be derived from the natural spring waters of certain regions, whether these were drunk, bathed in, or applied to the body in jets, douches, or poultices. The popularity of the mineral spring spas is indirectly related to the story of lithium.

The use of alkaline mineral waters was recommended for the treatment of mania by Soranus of Ephesus,[110] according to the translation of his works provided by Caelius Aurelianus in the fifth century.[111] In view of Soranus' further advice that the same alkaline waters should be employed for the relief of arthritis and similar complaints,[112] some early linking of affective disorders to more general physical disturbances can be seen: such an association was to find later expression in the idea of the uric acid diathesis of Garrod and Haig.

Whilst mineral springs had been noted for their medicinal properties long before the advent of Garrod and Haig,[113] it was in the late nineteenth century that there occurred a sudden and dramatic upturn in the fortunes of a large number of hydropathic establishments in various parts of the world. Although there were undoubtedly many economic and social reasons for this (better transport and communications, for example), it is nevertheless true that a major factor was the widespread support which the idea of the uric acid diathesis attracted, both from members of the medical profession and from the general public. The spas of Europe and North America became fashionable resorts for the wealthy who flocked to them in search of cures to the ailments, both real and imagined, to which the rich were, and are, particularly prone. Even those who could not afford to visit the mineral springs, or who could not do so as frequently as they might have wished, were nevertheless able to take advantage of the healing powers of the water by buying it in bottled form.

It was very much in the commercial interest of hydropathic centres and the distributors of bottled mineral water (both natural and specially prepared) to encourage, foster and maintain the idea put forward by Garrod and Lange that lithium salts – said to be present in the spring water – had beneficial effects in a large number of different disease states;[114] they were greatly aided in their task by the fact that Garrod himself had included in his recommended procedure for the treatment of gout, the drinking of mineral waters.

In 1887, Dr Willard Morse[115] was quite clear that what he saw as the undoubted advantages of natural mineral waters arose from an action upon excess uric acid by lithium salts which had a very 'long-deserved reputation for the cure of gout and rheumatism'.[116] He was also quick not only to deny the possibility of any deleterious effects arising from the waters but to emphasise the very wide range of conditions for which one might receive benefit. In the case of problems of the urinary tract, including calculi, prostatic enlargements, gonorrhoea, cystitis, stricture or acid urine, the waters would, he claimed, produce great relief, whilst in nephritis ' the water may be drunk *ad libitum*, with the assurance of cure in the early stages, and of palliation when the disease is advanced'.[117] There was, he added, no more potent remedy for Bright's disease. Incipient cirrhosis, portal vein congestion and jaundice were all said to respond well to lithia water which 'while it is not other than useless in hepatic colic ... has the property of preventing the attacks'.[118] The list of treatable conditions was virtually endless and included such diverse complaints as hepatic diabetes, obesity and atonic dyspepsia.

The *Lancet* of 1885 carried two accounts of the beneficial effects to be expected from certain French mineral springs, and a number of illuminating statements appear in them. Dr F. R. Cruise[119] reported to the Academy of Medicine in Ireland on visits which he had made to the springs at Contrexéville and Royat-les-Bains. He mentioned that Trousseau, an ardent proponent of the uric acid diathesis, was familiar with the internal use of Contrexéville waters and also that 'another disease in which Contrexéville water has been found very serviceable is diabetes ... certainly in the group of patients who are gouty',[120] suggesting that diabetes might be yet another condition assimilable into the uric acid (gouty) diathesis.[121] Elsewhere, Cruise remarked on the uses of the waters in diseases of the liver, 'especially those complicated by gall stones':[122] this is particularly interesting in view of a later use of lithium salts in the treatment of gall stones, a use which cannot be understood other than by an association of gall stones with renal stones, as seems to have been the case at Contrexéville.

Dr Cruise was himself a sufferer from a form of eczema, of which he wrote that, 'this affection, presumed from many special symptoms to be of a gouty nature, had been treated in various ways, but with very partial success'.[123] The waters of Royat-les-Bains, however, apparently succeeded where all else had failed. Yet another condition was added to the gouty diathesis. At Royat-les-Bains, the spring water was described as containing lithium chloride to the extent of 0.66 per cent of all solids in solution.

Dr Emile Emond, writing in the same issue of the *Lancet*[124] as Dr Cruise, reported on the successful treatment of bronchial asthma by the use of water from the springs of Mont Dore in the Auvergne. Dr Emond noted that Trousseau 'regarded asthma as a diathetic neurosis'.[125]

It would be possible to give accounts of very many more claims – literally hundreds – for the curative properties of spring waters and whilst each claim, taken alone, might be dismissed as inconclusive, relying on slender evidence and a confusion of many possible therapeutic factors, the sheer mass of evidence must have appeared almost overwhelming to the majority of medical practitioners of the late nineteenth century. There can be no doubt but that the successful assimilation of multifarious conditions into the uric acid diathesis, as well as the resilience of the concept of the diathesis itself, owed much to the vogue enjoyed by the mineral springs.

Lithium in mineral waters

That mineral springs might contain salts of lithium seems to have been first suggested by Berzelius in 1824 in reference to the waters of certain sources in Bohemia.[126] In 1839, Dr E. Osann[127] of Berlin gave details of the efficacy which might be expected of various lithium-containing waters in treating a number of urinary organ complaints; Alexander Ure was perfectly familiar with the work of Osann, to whom he referred as 'one of the latest and most complete writers on the subject',[128] and it is not unlikely that Ure drew the inspiration for his experimental work on the dissolution of uric acid as much from the writings of Osann on the subject of mineral springs as from those of Lipowitz.

Dr Burney Yeo, in 1888, reviewed the characteristics of a large number of European and British spas,[129] concluding that the water in the majority of them was likely to prove beneficial in individuals of a gouty constitution. That this benefit might derive from the presence of lithium salts in the spring waters was acknowledged by Yeo in his *Manual of Medical Treatment or Clinical Therapeutics*[130] in 1893, though he conceded that a number of writers had expressed considerable scepticism on the matter.

It did not take long for the mineral springs to come under close scrutiny by individuals with an interest in performing chemical analyses and the findings were, in all cases, unequivocal – the so-called lithia springs contained little lithium (and not infrequently none at all). Dr Frank L. James pointed out in 1889[131] that the figures given for the lithium content of commercially available bottled spring water were presented in a quite misleading way.[132] The following year, Dr E. Waller[133] made a careful analytic examination of several kinds of lithia water available in the USA. He could find no lithium at all in Farmville Lithia Water, and whilst in Buffalo Lithia Water lithium was present in detectable amounts, the actual concentration was 0.185 parts per million. Over twenty times richer was the third type of water, Londonderry Lithia Water, containing 4 parts per million. Of all the spring waters examined, the most concentrated had only 12 to 14 parts of lithium per million.

A similar exercise was carried out by Dr Charles Harrington of Harvard in 1896:[134] writing of the three most widely consumed lithia waters in the USA, he reported that he could find absolutely no lithium in two of them and no more than an unquantifiable trace in the third, concluding that 'two, by reason of excessive hardness, are not to be recommended for general household use; the other is a good water for all domestic purposes; not one can be said to be a medicinal water'.[135]

In 1910 Dr Henry Leffmann[136] reported the results of an investigation carried out by the United States Bureau of Chemistry, in the course of which forty-two so-called lithia waters commercially available in bottled form were analysed. Of these, twenty-one contained less than one hundreth of a grain of lithium per gallon; in seven there was less than 1 grain per gallon; only four possessed more than 2 grains per gallon and these contained so many other minerals and in such concentrations as to render them poisonous.

A delightful comment made by the Supreme Court of the District of Columbia related to a well-known lithia water:

> For a person to obtain a therapeutic dose of lithium by drinking Buffalo Lithia Water he would have to drink from one hundred and fifty thousand to two hundred and twenty-five thousand gallons of water per day. . . . Potomac River water contains five times as much lithium per gallon as the water in controversy.[137]

None of those who wrote about the low lithium content of spring waters actually raised serious objections to the general notion of the uric acid diathesis or to the claimed efficacy of lithium salts in its treatment. Indeed, they very often seemed at pains to assert otherwise. Dr James actually gave details of his own formula for a lithia water preparation in view of the fact that lithium salts had 'not only maintained the excellent impression which they first produced, but have continued to win a well-deserved reputation for certainty of action in a wide and constantly increasing field of therapeutics'.[138] Dr Harrington was only slightly less positive: 'pending an investigation of the question as to the real action of lithium salts,' he proposed, 'let it be conceded that these salts given in the usual doses produce the results claimed for them by recognised authorities'.[139] Leffmann felt uncertain enough of the claims for lithium for him to write that, 'the conclusion of the matter seems to me to be that it is doubtful if even lithium carbonate is of any real value in the treatment of lithiasis',[140] but he nevertheless suggested that the best way to obtain a high dose was by way of lithium tablets or by asking the local pharmacist to make up a lithium-containing drinking water.[141]

Alan Strobusch and James Jefferson, in a brief review of some aspects of the history of lithium therapy,[142] have related the appearance on the market of tablets for producing homemade lithium water to the fall from grace of the natural spring waters. The same may be true of the ready made-up lithia waters which began to appear around the turn of the century, but whilst the lithium tablets allowed at least a measure of control over the concentration of the resulting solution there was still considerable doubt about the precise therapeutic value of the concentrations existing in the ready-made bottled lithia waters, and occasionally legal proceedings were brought against the manufacturing companies. In 1908 the *Chemist and Druggist* carried a report[143] of just such a case brought before the Bournemouth Borough Bench in England against the Direct Supply Aerated Water Company. The lithia water sold by the company contained 1.2 grains of lithia per pint, the prosecution asserting that a concentration of eight times this was generally considered as standard. Dr J. A. Hosker, appearing for the defence said, however, that the lithia water contained sufficient lithia 'to constitute lithia water and to have an appreciable effect on the person drinking it'.[144] The case was dismissed.

Dr Jean Thuillier[145] has recalled a particular instance of proprietary lithia powder, used for making an effervescent drink – 'les lithinés du Dr Gustin':

Je me rappelle dans mon enfance, et certains d'entre vous aussi peut-être se rappelleront les lithinés du Dr Gustin.

On achetait dans les pharmacies des boites métalliques assez étanches, qui contenaient des sachets des poudre qu'il fallait mélanger à l'eau pour obtenir une boisson effervescente. On trouvait dans la boite, à côté des sachets, un petit entonnoir en carton qu'il fallait déplier et qu'on engageait dans le goulot d'une bouteille préalablement remplie d'eau. On faisait glisser, par l'entonnoir, la poudre contenue dans un sachet, on bouclait rapidement le bouteille qu'on basculait en l'agitant une ou deux fois. On voyait alors la poudre se dissoudre avec une effervescence qui parfois faisait sauter le bouchon de la bouteille s'il n'avait pas été bien enfoncé. Le breuvage ainsi preparé s'appelait un lithiné; il se buvait seul ou melangé au vin. Le prospectus de la boite disait qu'il était souvérain pour la goutte et les calculs urinaires, que le boisson était hygiénique et diététique et qu'on pouvait en user largement.

Assurement, à cette époque où nous ne disposions pas d'eaux minérales très gazeuses, la saveur piquante des lithinés du Dr Gustin était appreciée. Les indications du prospectus reposaient sur le fait que les sels de lithiné dissolvent les calculs urinaires formés par l'acide urique (urates). La lithiné était tout simplement de l'oxyde de lithium.[146]

Lithia pastilles, another form of concentrated lithia, were recorded in the literature as early as 1880.[147]

Doubts about the therapeutic value of lithium

It is, perhaps, remarkable that the uric acid diathesis, and certainly the therapeutic value of lithium, survived as viable medical ideas following the discrediting in the literature of the mineral springs. The fact that they not only survived but actually continued to have a most important influence on medical thought and practice over many subsequent years, attests to the durability of hypotheses advanced by those regarded as authorities in their field, to the lack of impact of scientific papers upon members of the general medical profession, and to the power of advertising by the manufacturers of lithia tablets and lithia water.

Not all clinicians were, however, fully convinced of the efficacy of lithium salts in the treatment of gout and some writers of the time were inclined to feel that Garrod might have been somewhat over-enthusiastic in his claim. In 1888, for example, Dr Burney Yeo,[148] whilst not contesting the value of lithium salts in absolute terms , expressed the opinion that they might have been overrated by comparison with other alkaline salts. Yeo noted that the alkaline salts in general might be expected to be effective in the treatment of the uric acid diathesis because of three kinds of action: by elevating blood alkalinity they would prevent acid urates being deposited; by their solvent actions they would help to remove existing urate deposits; and by promoting diuresis they would enhance uric acid elimination.

The employment of the salts of lithium for these purposes has acquired a wide publicity; for my own part, I am disposed to think we are, nowadays, inclined to exaggerate the value of the lithium compounds as compared with those of potash and soda. . . . When we are invited to select a mineral water for the treatment of these affections solely and especially because it contains, say, a tenth of a grain of chloride of lithium in a pint, in preference to another which contains 15 grains of bicarbonate of soda, we are running the risk of becoming the slaves of fashion.[149]

In 1883 Jahns[150] showed that lithium chloride added to distilled water failed to enhance the solubility of uric acid in the water, a result which was confirmed the following year, in the much more elaborate experiment, by Krumhoff.[151]

Other writers were also sceptical of the claims made for lithium salts in treating the uric acid diathesis. The *Chemist and Druggist* of 1860, for example, carried a brief article[152] on lithium and its salts in which, with rather heavy irony, reference was made to Garrod's 'elaborate treatise on gout, &c., in which complaint he attributes to carbonate of lithia wonderful and marvellous properties'.[153] A few years later, in the same journal, Dr Louis Siebold[154] stated quite explicitly that the high reputation of lithium salts for preventing the formation, or removing deposits, of uric acid was founded on very slim evidence. 'Altogether', he wrote, 'the superiority of lithia salts as remedies in calculus, gout, &c., appears to be very much over rated.'[155]

Mr C. W. Folkard was reported by the *Chemist and Druggist* of 1894[156] as characterising the lithium treatment of gout as an 'old but flourishing blunder in medicinal chemistry' and he concluded that 'the physician must in future look in another direction for a substance which will prove more advantageous in cases of uraemic poisoning.'[157]

The long life and slow death of the uric acid diathesis

The voices raised against the use of lithium for the treatment of conditions supposed to be related to uric acid metabolism, were relatively few and passed mostly unheeded. The uric acid diathesis concept was not only untouched, but went, indeed, from strength to strength. It had its staunch supporters who reacted strongly and effectively against the doubting faction.

An American physician, J. Lindsay Porteus, writing in the *New York Medical Journal* of 1893,[158] made a spirited defence of the uric acid diathesis: 'Some authorities', he wrote, 'state that there are no recognised symptoms of a definite kind to warrant the term "uric acid diathesis", but this I venture to question.'[159] He presented two case histories to illustrate his theme, and these are particularly interesting insofar as they confirmed that, by this time, mood disturbances were fully accepted as falling within the terms of the uric acid diathesis. The first patient, a ten-year-old girl, was described as being 'thin and neurotic' and 'often very bright and happy, but as often dull and depressed';[160] the second patient was a thirty-five-year-old man who, in addition to a great variety of other symptoms, showed 'a feeling of lassitude and drowsiness relieved by active exercise'.[161] Porteus argued that, in acid urine, uric acid was deposited and that an appropriate method of treatment therefore involved making the urine alkaline, for which purpose lithium salts had, he claimed. proved effective:

> In citrate of potassium we have a powerful agent to render the urine less acid, and, with the addition of benzoate of lithium, I have found in many cases that in from twenty-four to forty-eight hours I had neutralised the urine.[162]

By the end of the 1890s lithium salts were well-established as broad-spectrum treatments, not only in the eyes of the medical profession, but also by the general public – so much so, in fact, that Louis Kolipinski, a physician from Washington, was led to remark that:

since citrate of lithium in the form of effervescing tablets has come into popular use and is much employed by invalids for self-medication in a variety of ailments where lithia mineral water, in their judgement, seems indicated, I have thought it opportune to note that lithium salts are not innocuous bodies, and that they possess other than remedial properties.[163]

The uric acid diathesis became a major unifying principle in medical treatment to such an extent that it was possible in 1899 for a Danish physician, N. J. Strandgaard, to publish an extensive dissertation on gout and the uric acid diathesis,[164] in which he dealt with an enormous number of diseases which, in his view, could more or less reasonably be regarded as linked to the diathesis: these included diseases of the sensory, motor, vasomotor and secretory nerves, the central nervous system, the skin, the urinary and reproductive organs, the digestive system, the circulatory system, the respiratory system, the muscles and the sense organs. It seemed, in fact, that virtually any and every existing disease might be treated by prescribing a diet including alkaline mineral water and supplementary lithium salts, including the carbonate, salicylate, bromide, iodide, borate and benzoate.

Far from dying the rapid and total death which might have been expected of such a readily tested, and manifestly over-simplistic hypothesis, the uric acid diathesis concept clearly appears to have had astounding survival potential, and while it remained alive so too did the use of lithium salts.

The *Larousse Medical Illustré* of 1912[165] confirmed that the idea flourished at least until the beginning of the First World War. Alkaline salts, it pronounced, augmented urine secretion and dissolved renal and hepatic calculi as well as the tophi of gout:

Les principales maladies dans lesquelles on emploie les alcalins sont les maladies de l'estomac ... et du foie, la goutte, la gravelle, les coliques des reins, le muguet, les affections de la peau, le rhumatisme, la diathèse urique.[166]

Moreover, *Larousse Medical Illustré* subsumed under the general heading of 'arthritisme' such diverse illnesses as migraine, obesity, rheumatism, diabetes, asthma, emphysema, chronic gastritis, arteriosclerosis, hepatic colic, and renal gravel. Amongst the signs indicative of the onset of 'arthritisme' were listed a number of mental disorders, including apathy, agitation, extreme nervousness, emotional lability and sleep dysfunctions. Preventative measures which were proposed included open-air exercise and hydrotherapy, a number of mineral water spas being particularly recommended.

The use of lithium salts was extended to scrofula (lymph node tuberculosis), and although the rationale for this was not made clear, it was presumably related to the fact that potassium iodide was recommended for rheumatic diseases and that scrofula might manifest itself partly at the articular joints.[167]

The use of lithium salts to treat the uric acid diathesis survived even in the face of evidence that the solubility of uric acid was uninfluenced by the presence of lithium salts. For example, M. J. Moitessier[168] showed quite clearly in 1903 that neither the chloride nor the salicylate of lithium had the slightest effect on uric acid solubility. This work, was however, performed *in vitro* and was therefore open to the objection that in the more complicated *in vivo* situation, things might be quite different. Indeed, in 1914 experimental evidence was presented which seemed to support Garrod's proposal for using lithium salts to dissolve uric acid from deposits around joints. Amy L. Daniels, writing in the *Archives of Internal Medicine*,[169] argued that previous failure to demonstrate the dissolution of deposited urates *in vivo* might have been due to the saturation of the blood with uric acid prior to lithium administration and to an inability on the part of the kidneys to cope with such a situation; further solution of the deposited urates would therefore have no observable effect on excreted urate levels. Daniels suggested, however, that if kidney function could be enhanced to a point where the blood was no longer saturated with uric acid, then the action of lithium might be manifested. When atophan was used as a kidney function stimulator this did indeed appear to be the case, and Daniels concluded that 'in the absence of another reasonable explanation, the increase in the uric acid elimination when both atophan and lithium were being taken must be attributed to a solution of some of the deposited urates'.[170]

It is inevitable that such findings would help to maintain interest in the uric acid diathesis itself and in the use of lithium salts for treating the conditions related to the diathesis.

In 1924 Dr Hugo Weiss, an Austrian, reported[171] that lithium carbonate possessed therapeutic properties in diabetes. Whilst the claim was refuted in the same year by Professor S. Isaac[172] and Dr F. Depisch,[173] it is nevertheless of interest insofar as Dr Willard Morse[174] had spoken in 1887 of the close relationship between rheumatism and diabetes, and Garrod[175] himself had related diabetes to the uric acid diathesis: these considerations were, indeed, behind Weiss' claim.

Dr Malcolm Dyson, in the *Pharmaceutical Journal and Pharmacist* of 1931,[176] wrote that the bulk of lithium preparations found a use in pharmacy, their employment in this context depending upon the high solubility of lithium urate. In this article, only the slightest glimmer of doubt was expressed about the validity of the uric acid diathesis, the author merely permitting himself to wonder 'whether the effect [of lithium salts] on the progress of the gout is nearly so marked as the earlier investigators would have us believe'.[177]

As late as 1947 animal experiments were still being undertaken to check Garrod's suggestion that lithium salts should increase uric acid excretion. In France, Dr J. Mercier[178] gave both lithium campho-sulphonate and lithium benzoate to rabbits, but was unable to show uricolytic properties for either substance: the negative result is less interesting than the fact that anyone should still, in the middle of the twentieth century, have been contemplating the possibility that lithium might have an effect on uric acid metabolism.

In fact, there are many indications that the uric acid diathesis has found a niche in quite modern medical practice. One can even detect the residual influence of Alexander Ure's original findings: for example, in a medical textbook published in Germany in 1957,[179] it was indicated that oral lithium carbonate was still being recommended for the treatment of kidney and bladder stones; and René Hazard, in the 1956 edition of his authoritative textbook on pharmacology and therapeutics,[180] referred to the piperazine, lysidine, and anhydromethylene citrate of lithium as solvents of uric acid. John Talbott, in the second edition of his book, *Gout*,[181] which appeared in 1964, referred to 'the "gouty diathesis" which is still with us'.[182]

The Extra Pharmacopoeia and Merck's Index

The historical course of the introduction of various lithium compounds and preparations into pharmaceutical use as treatments for conditions subsumed under the uric acid diathesis, as well as the extraordinary persistence of the notion, is clearly seen by following the entries in successive editions of Martindale's *The Extra Pharmacopoeia*.

In the first edition,[183] which appeared in 1883, the bromide, carbonate and citrate were indexed, but only the first of these, the bromide, was dealt with in the body of the text: no medicinal properties were, however, indicated for the lithium ion, the compound being used for its properties as a bromide, presumably in the control of epilepsy.[184] The second edition[185] did, indeed, confirm that lithium bromide was 'a hypnotic, and to be used in epilepsy'.[186]

By the fourth edition (1885)[187] the text came to include the benzoate of lithium 'used as an anti-lithic',[188] and guaiacate of lithium 'given for chronic gout and rheumatism'.[189] It was Garrod[190] who had advocated the oral administration of guaiacum in association with alkaline salines to treat chronic gout: according to Garrod, guaiacum was effective in alleviating fibrous tissue problems. The association of guaiacum and lithium as lithium guaiacate was a quite logical extension of Garrod's ideas. It was also Garrod who had proposed the benzoates of both sodium and lithium in the treatment of uric acid deposits. Dr I. Burney Yeo, in an extensive address on the therapeutics of the uric acid diathesis, printed in the *British Medical Journal* in 1888,[191] noted that benzoic acid was held to prevent uric acid formation by combining with its precursor, glycosine, and appearing in the urine as hippuric acid. Yeo admitted himself to be unconvinced, though open-minded, as to the efficacy of the benzoates but noted their widespread use in France and Britain as remedies for excess uric acid formation.

The representation of lithium in the *Extra Pharmacopoeia* increased considerably three years later (1888) in the fifth edition,[192] to those compounds already listed being added the hippurate, which was described as a 'powerful solvent of lithates; useful in gout and rheumatism';[193] the salicylate (again for rheumatism and gout) and plaster of lithium-ichthyol which was applied to small wounds. It is not possible to say with any certainty what might be the origin of this topical use of lithium salts, although Garrod had himself suggested[194] that the external application of lithium carbonate might lead to the solution of gouty deposits and the alleviation of gouty inflammation, commenting, 'that it is of much value I do not entertain a doubt'.[195] There was, however, clear evidence that this was not so, Von G. Huffner[196] having demonstrated, in 1881, that lithium chloride solution applied to the feet for half an hour failed to find its way into the urine, even though the urine for a full 24-hour period was concentrated and submitted to spectroscopic analysis.

The introduction of lithium salicylate is explained by the fact that high doses of salicylates had been found to reduce blood levels of uric acid, hence heading off acute attacks of gout. In addition, Professor P. W. Latham[197] in 1885 had argued that rheumatic fever was caused by the excessive formation of glycosine and uric acid in the tissues and that salicylic acid prevented this by removing the metabolic antecedents and being then eliminated in the urine as salicyluric acid. Again, the combination of lithium and salicylic acid in the single salt, lithium salicylate, was an obvious step given prevailing views.[198]

As for lithium hippurate, the rationale for the inclusion of this salt would again appear to rest directly on the ideas of Garrod, who, in 1883[199], had pointed to the possible importance of hippuric acid[200] in nitrogen metabolism.

It was not until the eighth edition of *The Extra Pharmacopoeia* (1895)[201] that further additions occurred. Lithium tartrate was noted as being 'of special use in gouty cases with gum affections',[202] and 'Uricedin', 'a German speciality ... said to be prepared from concentrated lemon juice by treating it with sulphuric acid and hydrochloric acids, neutralised with soda, adding lithium citrate and evaporating to dryness',[203] was recommended for 'gout, gravel, urinary calculi, articular rheumatism, and uric acid diathesis'.[204] Uricedin was mentioned in 1893 by Dr M. Mendelsohn[205] in a paper directly concerned with the management of the uric acid diathesis and was regarded by Mendelsohn as being particularly suited to the long-term or prophylactic treatment of the diathesis.

The ninth edition (1898)[206] added lithium glycerophosphate, but without specifying its uses, though these were presumably by analogy with calcium glycerophosphate which was claimed to improve the 'general nutrition of the nervous system in all cases where nerve activity is enfeebled'.[207] One is led to speculate that the introduction of the lithium salt for such conditions may have followed the encompassing of nervous disorders into the uric acid diathesis.

In the same edition it was noted of lithium bromide that it was 'of great use in Bright's disease'.[208]

With the addition of varalettes of lithia to the list in the tenth edition in 1901,[209] a clear statement was made to the effect that 'the Lithium Salts do not exercise any special solvent action on sodium bi-urate, and are useless when given to remove uratic deposits';[210] despite this apparently unequivoc-al dismissal of lithium salts from any claim to therapeutic efficacy, The Extra Pharmacopoeia continued to recommend for use in gout, arthritis, rheumat-ism, and renal calculi, all those lithium salts previously indicated for such conditions in earlier editions. Moreover, by the eleventh edition (1904)[211] the statement had curiously disappeared, only to reappear two years later in the twelth edition[212] in a much less definite form, noting only that 'Lithium Salts have long had a reputation for assisting in the elimination of uric acid, but doubts are now felt on the subject'.[213] Again, in this edition, the individual compounds were characterised by the uses previously ascribed to them, with lithium iodide appearing as an anti-arthritic which was noted as having also been employed in the katophoretic (iontophoretic) treatment of syphilis. Lithium persulphate was suggested for rheumatism and gout.

It is likely that lithium iodide was introduced by analogy with potassium iodide, the latter having been employed since the early 1880s for the same conditions. Dr Burney Yeo, writing in 1888,[214] referred to the widespread use of potassium iodide in chronic arthritic affections 'but it has its most important applications, I believe, in the less easily recognised degenerative changes dependent on this diathesis'.[215].

The diuretic properties of lithium[216] which had been noted by Garrod and Mendelsohn amongst others, first made their appearance in The Extra Pharmacopoeia in its thirteenth edition (1908).[217] Lithium carbonate was described as a diuretic which increased the alkalinity of the blood; the citrate was also said to have diuretic properties. Lithium agaricinate was mentioned for the first time in this edition, being used 'to restrain the sweating of phthisis'.[218]

The fourteenth edition[219] saw the last appearance of Uricedin, and in the sixteenth edition of 1915[220] a warning was given about possible lithium poisoning following large doses of the chloride.[221] The use of lithium iodide was extended to the treatment of rheumatoid arthritis, according to the seventeenth edition (1922).[222]

An interesting change occurred in the eighteenth edition of The Extra Pharmacopoeia (1924)[223] in the wording of the statement expressing doubts about the effectiveness of lithium salts on uric acid. Their effect, it was stated, 'is probably analogous with corresponding potash salts'.[224] Despite this, the same treatment indications were repeated, and indeed not only was lithium bismutho-citrate added and noted as 'useful as a gout remedy',[225] but lithium phenyl-cinchoninate was specifically declared to be effective 'for elimination of uric acid, in acute and chronic gout'.[226]

It was not until the twenty-second edition, in 1941,[227] that *The Extra Pharmacopoeia* carried an unequivocal declaration that the reputation enjoyed by lithium salts for aiding uric acid elimination was ill-founded:

> Their introduction into medicine was due to a misconception . . . there is no rational foundation for the use of these salts.[228]

But, the note added, when given they should be freely diluted! Not only that, but the hippurate was still recorded as being used for gout and rheumatism, and the acid tartrate for gouty cases with gum affections.

All subsequent editions clearly and unequivocally indicated the lack of support for the use of lithium salts in conditions related to the uric acid diathesis. At the same time, a number of compounds originally introduced as antirheumatic agents (most remarkably, the salicylate, which first appeared in 1888) and for which no other possible use can be conceived, continued to be represented in the index of *The Extra Pharmacopoeia* as late as 1972 (the twenty-sixth edition).[229]

The Extra Pharmacopoeia provides a clear indication of the resilience of the uric acid diathesis and the consequent misuse in medical practice of lithium salts, well into the present century. A similar picture, though with some interesting variations, is provided by successive editions of *Merck's Index*, the first edition of which, published in 1889,[230] listed no fewer than twenty-nine lithium compounds and several lithium-containing mixtures. The third edition, of 1907,[231] presented a wide variety of lithium compounds, all the salts of lithium being, according to the *Index*, useful in lithiasis, arthritis and rheumatism and many were specifically indicated as effective against gout. In addition, the potential of lithium for alleviating various forms of mental distress (occurring in association with other conditions having a presumed aetiology involving excess uric acid) was indicated in a number of cases: the bromide was noted as being useful against headache in addition to its established uses in the treatment of epilepsy; lithium glycerinophosphate was recommended for the cure of gout accompanied by nervous debility; and lithium valerate was said to be efficacious against the hysteria and nervousness associated with rheumatism. The uric acid diathesis was several times mentioned in the 1907 edition.

The fourth edition of *Merck's Index* appeared in 1930[232] and was notable for the total acceptance which it displayed of both the uric acid diathesis and the efficacy of lithium against conditions falling within the diathesis. In this edition, compound after compound was described as having an antilithic action, as being anti-arthritic, antirheumatic, or antipodagric. Four compounds, the hippurate, iodate, iodide and oxalate, were specifically noted as being used for treatment of the uric acid diathesis. A number of rather curious uses were also listed for a few salts: lithium arsenate was said to be effective against skin disorders and anaemia; lithium benzoate, applied externally in aqueous solution, was used for removing calcareous spots in ulcerous corneal disease; lithium bitartrate was for pyorrhoea alveolaris; lithium bromide (in addition, of course, to its uses as an anti-epileptic and hypnotic) was prescribed for chronic parenchymatous nephritis; lithium oxalate was used to prevent blood coagulation; and lithium phenate was described as, amongst other things, an antiseptic. Various salts were said to be used in the manufacture of mineral waters, the carbonate being added to soda-water and lemonade.

Ten years later, in 1940, the fifth edition of *The Merck Index* appeared.[233] In many ways the entries resembled those of the fourth edition, but the words 'has been used in . . .' preceded most of the descriptions of the compounds' uses. However, lithium benzoate was still listed as useful for removing corneal calcareous deposits (a use based, presumably, on the supposed solubilising properties of lithium compounds) and the bromide was still said to be useful against nervous headache and hysteria. The chloride and carbonate were both, according to the *Index*, still being added to mineral waters.

By 1952, with the appearance of the sixth edition of the *Index*,[234] no therapeutic properties of any kind were ascribed to any lithium compound, though the chloride and citrate were both noted as occurring in mineral waters and soft drinks. The seventh edition (1960)[235] and the eighth (1968)[236] also gave this use for the same two compounds; and whilst in the ninth and latest edition (1976)[237] the citrate is recorded as no longer being used in soft drinks, the chloride is still said to be used in manufactured mineral waters.

It is clear, from both *The Extra Pharmacopoeia* and *The Merck Index* that whatever the theoretical status of the uric acid diathesis, it continued to exercise a considerable influence upon clinical therapeutics well into the second half of the twentieth century, as evidenced by the availability of a wide range of lithium compounds for the treatment of gout, arthritis, rheumatism and several other ailments.

Proprietary lithium-containing preparations

Despite the eventual disappearance from *The Extra Pharmacopoeia* and *The Merck Index* of references to the use of lithium salts in capacities related to the uric acid diathesis, the prescription of various lithium-containing mixtures in ways consistent with this concept nevertheless continued (and indeed continues) in a number of countries.

Uricedin, which disappeared from *The Extra Pharmacopoeia* in 1910,[238] could actually be obtained in West Germany over the counter and without prescription, until the early 1960s,[239] as could the Danish equivalent, Urisalin. This latter preparation, which contained lithium citrate and which was incorporated into the list of recipes for Danish pharmacists in 1906,[240] is still available, on prescription, in Denmark where its use in the recommended doses involves giving the patient between 12 and 17 millimoles of lithium per day.[241]

Also in Denmark, a lithium carbonate preparation with the name of Lithacyl, said to be indicated for rheumatic pains, neuralgia, influenza and menstrual discomfort, was available without prescription until 1965, and on prescription as late as 1971.[242]

In West Germany, Migrane-orotät, sold as tablets containing a considerable dose of lithium, was available at the end of 1980[243] and was described as useful for the treatment of migraine (a condition included by Garrod, Cantani and Haig in the rheumatic diathesis). At least twenty other lithium-containing products are currently obtainable in West Germany[244] (though the lithium content is, in general, quite low) and of these several are recommended as antirheumatics or as treatments for gout.

In Britain, too, most lithium compounds were available in proprietary preparations over the counter without prescription until the Medicine Act became law in February 1978. Some of these preparations were recommended for conditions formerly regarded as belonging to the uric acid diathesis. For example, Bishop's Gout Varalettes, containing lithium bitartrate, carbonate or citrate, were being sold by Alfred Bishop Ltd until 1976 when the company finally went out of business.[245] Ekner Tablets, containing lithium citrate and available prior to 1942 and up to about 1958, were labelled as an aperient and diuretic useful in cases of constipation associated with rheumatic conditions; Ekner Powder, of similar constitution to the tablets and available at about the same time, carried a claim on the label to be three-in-one health salts for attractive good health, antacid and special laxative, for pep, vitality, enthusiasm and endurance and further asserted itself to be a brain, body and stomach restorer.

A rather curious extension of the uric acid diathesis is to be found in a lithium-containing preparation available in Finland in 1940: *Tinctura zedoariae compositae*, containing lithium benzoate, was described as *sappikivitipat* or 'gall stone drops'.[246] It would appear that the use of lithium salts for the dissolution of kidney stones, as proposed by Alexander Ure, had been transferred, without any logical medical reason, to the treatment of gall stones, and this also recalls the use of certain mineral springs for the cure of liver disorders characterised by gall stones.[247]

A lithium preparation called Rheumin pulv., sold as an antirheumatic, was available without prescription in Finland until 1967.[248]

In Israel at the present time a preparation called Urisolvine granules is available on prescription for the treatment of kidney stones.[249] This mixture contains, in addition to five other ingredients, 0.2 per cent of lithium carbonate.

It is certain that a survey of other countries would reveal a wealth of lithium-containing preparations available for treating ailments once subsumed under the uric acid diathesis.

Influence of the uric acid diathesis

All those who dismiss the idea of the therapeutic properties of lithium against uric-acid-related disorders, as being founded upon a misconception, are still faced with the necessity of explaining why it was that some early investigators actually found changes in uric acid excretion apparently resulting from lithium administration. Could it simply be that the experimental techniques were so crude that gross errors were made? Surely the findings could not have resulted from over-enthusiastic interpretation of the data?

Some light was shed on this problem in 1968 when a group of investigators[250] from the University of Edinburgh re-examined the influence of lithium treatment on uric acid metabolism in manic–depressive patients and did indeed find that uric acid excretion was elevated following administration of lithium carbonate. Interpretation of this was complicated by the finding that increased excretion of uric acid was also associated with spontaneous recovery without lithium. However, the size of the lithium-induced excretory response was sufficiently great to persuade the investigators that a real effect of lithium occurred, over and above that explicable by therapeutic improvement and by increased diuresis. Whilst the findings were interpreted in terms of lithium-produced alterations of organic acid active-transport in the kidney, and not as justifying the theoretical basis of the uric acid diathesis, the work is interesting insofar as it renders explicable the nineteenth century linking of lithium and uric acid metabolism.

The history of the uric acid (arthritic, rheumatic, gouty) diathesis becomes of particular interest in the wider context of contemporary psychiatric usage of lithium salts if it can be established that the pioneers of modern lithium therapy were either aware of, or were influenced – perhaps indirectly – by the ideas advanced by Ure, Garrod, Haig and others. The evidence for this is difficult to establish, often equivocal, and almost always circumstantial, but such evidence as does exist will be reviewed in later chapters.

One thing, however, is certain, and that is that the therapeutic effectiveness of lithium salts in the treatment of affective disorders was well known to nineteenth-century physicians, even though such applications were based upon quite erroneous premises. The resilience of the discredited uric acid diathesis in the face of very clear contrary evidence is a matter for some reflection, but whatever the forces which were at work to preserve the potency of the concept, the net result was to ensure that a considerable variety of lithium salts was always readily available to the physician – a fact which, in all probability, facilitated the subsequent incorporation of such substances into medical practice when the time was ripe.

3

The work of John Cade

The early experimental studies

John Frederick Joseph Cade was born on 18 January 1912 at Horsham, a small country town in Victoria, Australia. Like his father before him, John Cade entered the medical profession, obtaining his MB, BS (Melbourne) in 1934. After a period during which he held a residency first at a general hospital and then at a hospital for children, he took up a position in 1936 with the mental health services of Victoria. Two years later, in 1938, he obtained his MD (Melbourne).

During the Second World War, he rose to the rank of Major in the 2/9th Field Ambulance (Eighth Division), but was captured by the Japanese and held as a prisoner of war for three and a half years.

It was, according to his own report,[1] during this time in the prison camp that his ideas on the physiological basis of mental disorders gradually took shape:

> I could see that so many of the psychiatric patients suffering from the so-called functional psychoses appeared to be sick people in the medical sense. This fired my ambition to discover their etiology. . . . I returned from three and a half years as a POW of the Japanese mourning the wasted years and determined to pursue the ideas that had germinated in that interminable time.[2]

The basis of these ideas lay in his feeling that mania might represent a state of intoxication arising as a result of an excess of some normal metabolite, whilst depression represented the effects of abnormally low levels of the same metabolite.

When, on New Year's Day 1946, John Cade resumed his psychiatric work (at the Repatriation Hospital, Bundoora – an outer suburb of Melbourne) he immediately set to work to devise a method whereby the existence of the hypothesised metabolite might be demonstrated.

Inevitably, the work was technically primitive. One of John Cade's sons (also called John, and also a doctor) has some recollections[3] of the early days of the research:

> Although I was only about nine years old at the time, I remember that the work was carried out in the pantry of a still vacant new ward that had been built at Bundoora Hospital after the Second World War. There was only a bench, sink, a few jars of chemicals, some simple lab instruments (pipettes etc.) and the guinea-pigs. These were housed in our back garden and looked after as family pets.[4]

John Cade himself acknowledged[5] the crudity of the investigations and the vagueness of the underlying hypothesis.

> Because I did not know what the substance might be, still less anything of its pharmacology for lower animals, the best plan seemed to be to spread the net as wide as possible and use the crudest form of biological test in a preliminary investigation.[6]

> The only solution seemed to be to devise an extraordinarily crude differential toxicity test and discover whether any differentials emerged. And crude it was.[7]

Early-morning urine samples, passed after abstinence from fluids for 12–14 hours were collected from manic, depressive and schizophrenic patients as well as from normal control subjects. The urine was then injected intraperitoneally into the guinea-pigs. That from the manic patients proved to be far more toxic than from the other groups, although all samples led to deaths amongst the animals. As Cade put it:

> All that had been demonstrated so far was that any concentrated urine in sufficient quantity would kill a guinea-pig, but that urine from a manic subject often killed much more readily.[8]

The sequence of events leading up to the death of the guinea-pigs was identical for all urine samples, suggesting that the toxic principle was the same in each case. The toxicity was traced to urea which, in large doses, produced death in the same way as the patients' urine. There were, however, two problems for Cade: the first was that none of the urine samples differed from any of the others in terms of the urea concentration; and the second was that the urea concentration in all cases was far below the toxic minimum. To overcome this difficulty, Cade suggested that there might exist what he called 'quantitative modifiers', that is to say other substances which, by their presence, enhanced the toxic effects of urea. In fact, Cade postulated two such substances: creatinine, which affected urea toxicity negatively, giving protection against its poisonous action; and uric acid which had a positive effect, enhancing urea toxicity (but still not sufficiently to account for the lethal effect of patients' urine in guinea-pigs). Cade was forced to propose that a third, unidentified, substance might 'neutralise' the protective effect of creatinine. The model became unwieldy at this point and Cade turned his attention to investigating further the effects of uric acid on urea toxicity. Again a problem was encountered:

> The practical difficulty was the comparative insolubility of uric acid in water, so the most soluble urate was chosen – the lithium salt. And that is how lithium came into the story.[9]

However, with lithium urate, urea was *less*, not more, toxic than it was when administered alone. This was a surprising result given Cade's earlier finding that uric acid had either no effect or produced a slight enhancement of urea toxicity, and it seemed that the lithium ion may have given some degree of protection against urea toxicity. To check this, lithium carbonate was used instead of the urate, with identical effects. Finally, to discover whether lithium salts used alone produced effects on guinea-pigs, 'large doses'[10] of a 0.5 per cent aqueous carbonate solution were administered intraperitoneally to the animals. The results were of historic importance:

> after a latent period of about two hours the animals, although fully conscious, became extremely lethargic and unresponsive to stimuli for one to two hours before once again becoming normally active and timid.[11]

To this description, Cade later added:

> Those who have experimented with guinea-pigs know to what extent a ready startle reaction is part of their make-up. It was thus even more startling to the experimenter to find that after the injection of a solution of lithium carbonate they could be turned on their backs and that, instead of their usual frantic righting behaviour, they merely lay there and gazed placidly back at him.[12]

It is more than probable that the behavioural effects which Cade observed were so marked because the lithium dose was in the toxic range. The American psychiatrist Nathan Kline[13] has raised just this point, but concluded that:

> If we were to eliminate from science all great discoveries that had come about as the result of mistaken hypotheses or fluky experimental data, we would be lacking half of what we know (or think we know).[14]

Certainly Cade could hardly have failed to have known that lithium salts were associated with some toxic effects in view of the work of one or two earlier experimenters such as Good[15] and Cleaveland,[16] but he seems not to have been aware of a number of contemporary studies claiming serious toxicity and even fatalities as a result of lithium salt ingestion.[17] Nevertheless, before using lithium to treat patients, Cade tried it out on himself:

> How to proceed? *Primum non nocere.* The older pharmacopoeias did not describe any toxic effects of lithium salts but was that good enough? There is always the number one experimental animal, oneself.[18]

Again the investigation was home-based. John Cade's son records:

> Our kitchen refrigerator usually had jars of manic patients' urine and racks of blood samples in it, always on the top shelf and much to my mother's consternation. Her greatest distress came when Dad started taking lithium carbonate himself for a few weeks before giving it to patients.[19]

The first clinical trial

Concluding that lithium was without serious untoward effects, Cade embarked on what was the first clinical trial of lithium, though by modern standards it left much to be desired in the way of design and methodology. Either the citrate or the carbonate were used – the former because of its solubility, the latter because of its lower tendency to produce gastric disturbances. In some of his later writings, Cade gives the impression that the dose levels of the two salts were apparently chosen at random:

> The original therapeutic dose decided on fortuitously proved to be the usual optimum, that is 1200 mg of the citrate or 600 mg of the carbonate thrice daily.[20]

In fact, the decision on dosage was rather more thoughtful and based upon a consideration of values given in the *British Pharmacopoeia* and a number of textbooks of materia medica.[21]

In the 3 September 1949 issue of the *Medical Journal of Australia* (just ten years after the start of the Second World War, as Cade used to point out[22]) an article appeared in which Cade outlined the results of his clinical trial.[23] He gave details of ten patients, three of whom were described as showing chronic mania, the rest having mania in an episodic form. In fact, from the clinical description, at least one of the patients showing recurrent mania was probably manic–depressive, and one might nowadays be classed as schizo-affective.

The findings appeared to be dramatic. In all cases, lithium was reported to have reduced psychotic excitement, the clinical symptoms returning on the withdrawal of lithium. In addition, six schizophrenic patients also showed some reduction in excitement (restlessness, noisiness, etc.) but not in their fundamental schizophrenic pathology (hallucinations, thought disorder). Three chronically depressed patients failed to respond to lithium though no worsening of their condition was reported.

Cade concluded that lithium possessed a specific antimanic action, and hazarded a guess about 'the possible aetiological significance of a deficiency in the body of lithium ions in the genesis of this disorder';[24] his proposal that lithium might be an essential trace element has not, however, received any support from subsequent work.

Cade's descriptions of his individual manic patients are particularly interesting. In the first place, cases of chronic mania such as he treated are nowadays very rarely found in hospitals, and secondly, they reveal Cade's particularly thoughtful approach to lithium treatment. For example, the patient described as T.F. was actually taken off lithium when it was realised that despite the elimination of manic behaviour there was constant abdominal discomfort and even when no longer manic he was still a mildly enfeebled, irritable old man.

Similar considerations applied in the first case reported; this patient, W.B., was regarded by Cade as the one in which lithium treatment was eventually most successful, though there were initial difficulties in getting the treatment established.

> The very first manic patient ever deliberately and successfully treated with lithium salts . . . was a little wizened man of 51 who had been in a state of chronic manic excitement for 5 years. He was amiably restless, dirty, destructive, mischievous and interfering. He had enjoyed pre-eminent nuisance value in a back ward for all those years and bid fair to remain there for the rest of his life. He commenced treatment with lithium citrate 1200 mg thrice daily on 29 March 1948. On the fourth day, the optimistic therapist thought he saw some change for the better but acknowledged that it could have been his expectant imagination (it was April Fool's Day!). The nursing staff were non-committal but loyal. However, by the 5th day it was clear that he was in fact more settled, tidier, less disinhibited and less distractible. From then on there was steady improvement so that in 3 weeks he was enjoying the unaccustomed and quite unexpected amenities of a convalescent ward. As he had been ill so long and confined to a closed chronic ward he found normal surroundings and liberty of movement strange at first. Owing to this, as well as housing difficulties and the necessity of determining a satisfactory maintenance dose, he was kept under observation for a further 2 months.

He remained perfectly well and left hospital on 9 July 1948, on indefinite leave, with instructions to take a maintenance dose of lithium carbonate 300 mg twice daily.

The carbonate had been substituted for the citrate as he had become intolerant of the latter, complaining of severe nausea. He was soon back working happily at his old job.

It was with a sense of the most abject disappointment that I readmitted him to hospital 6 months later as manic as ever but took some consolation from his brother who informed me that Bill had become overconfident about having been well for so many months, had become lackadaisical about taking his medication and had finally ceased taking it about 6 weeks before. Since then he had become steadily more irritable and erratic. His lithium carbonate was at once recommenced and in 2 weeks he had again returned to normal. A month later he was recorded as completely well and ready to return to home and work.[25]

In addition, Cade's original and hitherto unpublished clinical notes[26] on the case of W.B., make it clear that considerable problems were encountered in respect of side effects, particularly dyspepsia, vomiting and bradycardia. Lithium was discontinued and recommenced on several occasions. The last occasion of discontinuation was on 8 February 1950, when Cade wrote in his notes:

Lithium discontinued. Under all the circumstances it seems that he would be better off as a carefree case of mania rather than the dyspeptic, frail little man he looks on adequate lithium.[27]

By 28 March, W.B. was recorded as reverting to his manic phase and losing his dyspepsia, but on 12 May Cade wrote:

Has continued manic – restless, euphoric, noisy, dirty, mischievous, destructive, flight of ideas. This state seems as much a menace to life as any possible toxic effects of Li. [Therefore] recommenced *Li cit* today.[28]

In fact, W.B. subsequently died of lithium toxicity,[29] but not before he had shown a dramatic recovery from his chronic state of mania.

An interesting sidelight on patient W.B. is that Cade recorded in his original clinical notes an extraordinarily high value for blood uric acid level just over three weeks before commencing treatment with lithium citrate,[30] noting that 'this extremely high blood uric acid result is suspect'.[31]

Problems revealed in the original case notes

In several of the cases as reported in the *Medical Journal of Australia* there are minor, but interesting, variations from the clinical case notes. Case VI, referred to as A.M., was recorded in the published article[32] as being put on a maintenance dose of 10 grains of lithium citrate one week after commencing the therapeutic dose on 14 February 1949; in the case notes, however, the entry for 21 February reads: 'refuses to take Li_2CO_3'.[33]

Case VIII (W.M.) was described as 'practically normal – quiet, tidy, rational, with insight into his previous condition'[34] after two weeks on lithium citrate which had commenced on 11 February 1949. The original case notes extend beyond this date and record evident lithium toxicity (ataxia) leading to temporary withdrawal of medication on 1 March[35] and then to a resumption of the maintenance dose on 5 March.[36] Lithium was finally withdrawn on 10 April, the patient complaining of anorexia, unsteadiness, general malaise and depression.[37]

The published account[38] of case IX (W.S.) ends by noting that 'he recommenced taking lithium citrate 10 grains twice a day on 4 March 1949. An acquaintance who has known the patient for years reports that he has never seen him as normal as at present'.[39] This parallels the entry for 4 March[40] in the case notes, but there are two further entries: the first of these indicates that six days later W.S. had become 'rather garrulous' and that the dose of lithium citrate was thus increased;[41] the second entry, on 15 March,[42] notes that he was still garrulous and had diarrhoea. Lithium was then discontinued.

Cade never mentioned, in any of the published accounts of his work, the fact that his first patient (case I, W.B.) died of lithium poisoning. It is worth looking at the later stages of this case in some detail. Almost two years after first taking lithium, W.B. was readmitted to hospital. According to Cade's notes for 8 February 1950,[43] W.B. had been feverish over the preceding week, with dyspepsia, nocturnal vomiting and diarrhoea. There was some bradycardia. His mental state, however, was good, and he was returned to the hostel where he was boarding. One month later[44] he still seemed quite well mentally but the bradycardia persisted. Dyspepsia disappeared following a dosage reduction in the lithium carbonate. He was then taken off lithium carbonate altogether. Two months later W.B. was 'back to his old form again – restless, dirty, mischievous, destructive and thoroughly pleased with himself'.[45] He remained in this state for just over a week, becoming emaciated and developing infected, self-inflicted sores, so the decision was then taken to resume lithium treatment.[46] The treatment started to calm W.B. almost immediately, but within a week[47] the lithium was again withdrawn since W.B. became semi-comatose and had three fits just after midday. By 4.30 that afternoon he was being tube fed, and although looking rather better was still only semiconscious. On 22 May,[48] Cade recorded that W.B. was 'in extremis' at 9.00 a.m. His skin was 'breaking down everywhere' and there was continuous myoclonic twitching. Despite a temporary slight improvement, W.B. died at 11.15 p.m. the following day.[49] Cade recorded as the primary cause of death 'toxaemia due to lithium salts therapeutically administered'[50] and noted that, in view of this, the case had been reported to the coroner.

These discrepancies between case records and published accounts, though fairly slight, are probably not unimportant, in that they combined to make the published account rather more favourable to lithium than would have been the case had the clinical case records been adhered to rather more closely. It would, however, be quite unfair to suggest that Cade was being deliberately misleading: he was, indeed, very candid in other parts of his article concerning the toxic effects of lithium and he did not attempt to underplay the need for very careful monitoring of the treatment:

> The symptoms of over-dosage are referable mainly to the alimentary and nervous systems. Abdominal pain, anorexia, nausea and vomiting occur and occasionally mild diarrhoea. The nervous symptoms are giddiness, tremor, ataxia, slurring speech, myoclonic twitching, asthenia and depression. The patient looks ill – pinched, drawn, grey and cold.
> Unless such symptoms are followed by immediate cessation of intake there is little doubt that they can progress to a fatal issue. It is therefore of the utmost importance that when a patient is on maximum doses he should be seen each day and that the nursing staff should be instructed to look for early symptoms of intoxication.[51]

Nevertheless, therapeutic advantages and toxic side effects were fairly sharply demarcated in the published report (side effects being mentioned only thirteen times in all and none at all being reported for five of the patients, as distinct from forty-one mentions in the clinical records) and this must undoubtedly have enhanced the chances that the findings would be taken seriously. In fact, Cade made a note in his personal case records of the majority of the side effects and toxic symptoms which were later to be reported for lithium by other investigators and had he dwelt upon these at greater length than he actually did, it is doubtful whether his work would have been accorded more than a passing consideration.

There is evidence that Cade was deeply troubled by the toxic side effects of lithium, to an extent which did not communicate itself in print. Samuel Gershon, who was working in Melbourne at the time that Cade was doing his early experiments and treating his first patients, records that Cade was sufficiently anxious about the possibility of serious poisoning that he discontinued lithium treatment.

> Investigations into the specific properties of the lithium ion itself were first carried out by Cade in 1949, only to be abandoned because of lithium toxicity.[52]

The last of the survivors of the original ten manic patients (patient V, B.D.) died in 1980, at the age of 76, of a massive heart attack,[53] after more than thirty years on lithium treatment, and in the same year that saw the death of the man who had restored him to health.

Treatment of schizophrenia

In 1969, Cade gave a brief report[54] of two schizophrenic patients who had been treated with lithium by Dr Chesler, one of Cade's colleagues at the Royal Park Psychiatric Hospital in Melbourne. Both patients responded well, and although the brief case descriptions suggest that the lithium effect was probably on the affective components of a schizo-affective syndrome, Cade commented that 'psychiatrists often argue fruitlessly about the diagnosis when confronted by atypical reactions. It is far more important to ask not whether a psychotic reaction is manic or schizophrenic, but rather whether it is likely to be a lithium-responsive psychosis'.[55]

Serendipity?

It has frequently been said that Cade's discovery of the antimanic action of lithium was the result of pure chance – 'serendipitous' is a word frequently used[56] – but Cade himself always insisted that this was not so, and that the sequence of steps from his first experiments on urine injected into guinea-pigs, to the administration of lithium salts to manic patients, was completely logical and understandable. Any suggestion that the discovery was other than the result of a clearly defined chain of reasoning caused Cade great irritation:

> People inevitably ask why lithium should have been tried in the treatment and prophylaxis of affective illness and especially, in the first place, of manic episodes. It is, of course, a perfectly valid question. Why not try potable pearl, or crocodile dung or unicorn horn? I was asked by a reporter some years ago – I thought rather unkindly – whether I had discovered it whilst shaving one morning.
> It is naturally the profoundest mystery unless one is aware of the preceding and intermediate steps. Then it can be seen, with such hindsight, to have been the almost inevitable result of experimental work I was engaged in, in an attempt to elucidate the aetiology of manic–depressive illness.[57]

Cade's later work

After his initial work on lithium, John Cade did little more in the way of original research, though over the ensuing years he undertook a series of rather slight investigations involving other metallic ions.[58] It was, he said, inevitable 'having thus been unexpectedly presented with a therapeutic magic wand, that one would plunge one's hand time and again into the same lucky dip'.[59] He looked at rubidium and caesium, both of which he found to be without effect in either guinea-pigs or rats. Cerium salts, though producing marked sedative effects in rats, had no psychopharmacological action in man; similar results were noted for lanthanum and neodymium, but praesodymium failed to affect even the rats. Strontium salts, he claimed, had marked anxiolytic properties, and after trying it out on himself (it had a tranquillising action), he tested it clinically.

As it had a tranquillising and mildly sedative effect on such a relatively pharmacologically tough animal as myself, it seemed reasonable to evaluate it further, and over 10 months its effects on over 30 patients suffering from a variety of psychiatric disorders was assessed. There is no doubt whatever that it is substantially anxiolytic, safe, effective, and cheap. Even in patients who showed no real improvement otherwise, there was in many cases a tranquillising effect with diminished restlessness and in some, drowsiness. In the two patients with anxiety severe enough to warrant hospitalisation, there was complete and prompt remission in two days. In seven acute schizophrenics there was complete and prompt remission in four, substantial symptomatic improvement in another, and in two no effect whatever....

Most would agree that this is tenuous evidence on which to base any sort of therapeutic claim and I wholeheartedly concur. I merely present the results as interesting, possibly significant, certainly worthy of further study.[60]

The lead was not followed, however, and lithium therapy was to remain the sole legacy of John Cade's experimental work.

Cade and the uric acid diathesis

When Cade undertook the work which was to lead to the rediscovery of lithium therapy, uric acid again entered the story. In considering the most likely candidate for his hypothetical enhancer of urea toxicity, he went immediately to uric acid and thence to the most soluble of the uric acid salts – lithium urate. Although Cade did not see his work as a progression from the ideas of Haig, Lange and the rest of the proponents of the uric acid diathesis, no research worker is ever truly free of the influences of his scientific forbears. Cade was clearly aware of Garrod's writings and quoted Garrod's authority for supposing lithium urate to be the most soluble of the urates. Is it possible that Cade's immediate choice of uric acid as the putative modifier of urea toxicity owed its spontaneity to the still current (or, at least, very recently deceased) uric acid diathesis concept?

Having found that not only lithium urate, but lithium carbonate too, produced effects on guinea-pigs Cade unhesitatingly transferred his attentions to hospitalised patients. Why was he so positive in taking such a decision? Did he have any reason, other than the results of his guinea-pig studies, for believing that a successful outcome in his patients was likely? Probably not – at least not in a formal, explicit way; but it seems hardly likely that the various claims which had been put forward for over a hundred years for the therapeutic benefits of lithium in a wide range of disorders, including mental affections, were either totally unknown to Cade or failed to influence his thought, at least in a general way.

At the time that he published his first account of lithium treatment for psychotic excitement John Cade was Senior Medical Officer in the Department of Mental Hygiene of Victoria, Australia, and it is at this point that a further[61] curious coincidence appears in the lithium story. In February 1903, the Brecon and Radnor Asylum (now the Mid-Wales Hospital) at Talgarth, Wales, appointed as its first Medical Superintendent Dr W. Ernest Jones. The appointment was relatively brief, for at the end of 1904 Dr Jones left the Mid-Wales Hospital to take up a position described by the 1905 Report of the Commissioners in Lunacy as 'Inspector General of Insane for the Colony of Victoria'.[62] There is some evidence to suggest that Dr Jones may have employed lithium during his time at the Mid-Wales Hospital: a later Superintendent to the same hospital, Dr Gordon Diggle, who took over responsibility in 1948, recalls having found a large seven- or fourteen-pound canister of a lithium salt (carbonate or citrate – probably the latter) in the hospital dispensary; the canister bore a label which, by its style of printing, dated it to the early years of the century.[63] Dr Diggle, noting that the large canister was half empty, has suggested that such large quantities of a lithium salt were unlikely to have been used to prepare lithia water but 'must have been used for psychiatric illness'[64] – a conclusion made the more probable since the hospital dealt exclusively with psychiatric patients. The canister no longer exists: Dr Diggle disposed of it in 1948.

Did Dr Jones take with him to Victoria a belief that lithium might, for whatever reason, be effective in treating certain types of mental illness? If he did, then were such ideas still 'in the air' when John Cade came to Victoria just over 40 years later?[65]

The thought has certainly occurred to others. Dr Amdi Amdisen of Denmark, for example, has commented that, 'it seems ... very probable that the senior doctors at his [Cade's] mental hospital during the late forties may have known about lithium as an antidepressant drug in their younger days'.[66]

There is no doubt that lithium compounds *were* available for medicinal use in Australia well before John Cade did his experimental work.[67] In 1940, for example, a wide variety of lithium salts were listed in various pharmaceutical compendia, for purposes which included the treatment of arterial hypertension and of gastric acidity, and the induction of diuresis.[68] Cade would certainly have had no difficulty at all in obtaining supplies of lithium salts from the dispensary of the hospital in which he worked, thanks to the continuing influence of the uric acid diathesis.

John Cade's place in the history of lithium therapy

Whether one regards John Cade as the discoverer or the rediscoverer[69] of the effectiveness of lithium in the treatment of affective disorders, is really of very little consequence when it comes to determining the role which he played in laying the foundations of modern lithium therapy. It is certain that, without his work, modern psychiatry would have had to wait for many more years to gain this most valuable therapeutic tool – and might, indeed in all probability, still have been waiting.

The way in which the scientific community receives a new idea is very much dependent upon how that idea is promulgated by the person who first puts it forward. Whilst a certain amount of circumspection is both expected and appropriate, it is nevertheless necessary that the idea should be projected enthusiastically, forcefully and, above all, frequently, if maximum impact is to be achieved: modesty is not a quality which contributes a great deal to success in establishing the idea and its originator in the forefront of scientific debate. John Cade was a modest man. His scientific writings were economical – often blunt – in their style, making no use of special pleading or hyperbole. When, in the last few years of his life, he wrote a short, but hugely entertaining, book[70] dealing with his own very personal view of the history of twentieth-century psychiatry, he included a long section on the discovery and use of lithium therapy without once identifying himself as the discoverer.[71]

John Cade was a scientist in the classical mould – an enquirer with catholic interests and the intellectual courage to attempt to answer fundamental questions by means of relatively simple techniques. One day he may well be generally recognised as ranking amongst the most influential figures of twentieth-century psychiatry.

4

The toxicity panic

At the time that John Cade published his discovery of the therapeutic effects of lithium salts, psychiatric practice was ripe for acceptance of powerful, new, drug-based treatment procedures. Advances in biology in the first half of the century had led to a movement away from the almost purely descriptive, taxonomic approach which was the legacy of nineteenth-century preoccupation with natural history, towards a more functional, mechanistic orientation. It was no longer acceptable simply to say *how* organisms functioned or were constructed; it was necessary also to provide some kind of answer to the question of *why* – in terms of biochemical or physiological processes – an organism functioned or was structured in one way rather than another. In short, the emphasis was upon *control* processes. Questions of how *normal* functions were controlled, quickly led to the related and, from the clinical scientist's point of view, much more interest-ing, question of how abnormal processes arose and could be modified – reversed, even – by outside intervention aimed at influencing the aberrant or dysfunctional control processes underlying the pathological abnormality.

That something of the kind was possible, both in principle and in practice, had long been known. Certain pharmacological interventions were already quite widely accepted and used: the barbiturates, for example, had been introduced into medical practice as early as 1903 when Fischer and Von Mering[1] succeeded in synthesising barbital, whilst the stimulant properties of the amphetamines were recognised some twenty-five years later and led to this group of drugs being extensively employed against depression and other retarded behavioural states.[2] Even before the barbiturates were accepted as important sedatives and anxiolytics, there were other substances which had been adopted in this capacity: the bromides were first used as anti-epileptic agents in 1857 and the hypnotic effects of chloral hydrate were recognised shortly afterwards, in 1869; paraldehyde, another hypno-tic, was introduced around 1884.[3]

When chlorpromazine became available in the early 1950s it was seized upon by psychiatrists with an avidity and enthusiasm the like of which had seldom previously been seen in medical practice. Certainly, by the middle of the twentieth century the general atmosphere in clinical psychiatry was as receptive as it had ever been to the introduction of pharmacological treatment procedures.

The big problem with all the available medications, including chlorpromazine, was that they were relatively nonspecific in their effects, and whatever therapeutic potential they possessed could often be ascribed merely to an overall suppressant or stimulant action which blanketed or masked the pathological symptoms – and did so, moreover, along with similar, and quite unwanted, effects on a range of normal functions too. When Cade showed that lithium could eliminate mania without apparently affecting schizophrenic processes at the same time, it looked as though here was the first specific pharmacological treatment ever discovered in the field of psychiatry.[4]

One might therefore have reasonably expected that the news about lithium would have been received with considerable interest, both by those engaged in developing theories concerning the biological bases of abnormal behaviour and particularly by those engaged in treating such behaviour. That this did not happen – that, on the contrary, lithium was generally ignored by all but a few individuals and groups[5] – is a matter which clearly needs explanation. The answer is, in fact, relatively simple: lithium salts proved to be poisonous.

The case of the substitute salt

In 1936, *The Extra Pharmacopoeia*[6] carried a brief note to the effect that lithium chloride had a salty taste, a fact which, given the chemical similarity to sodium chloride, was not altogether unexpected. This property led to lithium chloride being used as a major constituent of a number of salt substitutes developed in the USA and first marketed in 1948. Four main brands of salt substitute – Westsal,[7] Foodsal, Salti-salt and Milosal – became available to the general public and were immediately very widely used. In particular, they were recommended by doctors to patients suffering from hypertension, cardiac disease or renal disease with oedema, and for whom a diet containing little or no sodium chloride was appropriate: such diets often seemed dull and uninteresting, and the addition of a substance possessing a salt taste whilst lacking the adverse physiological properties of sodium chloride, made meals more palatable.

The salt substitutes were often in the form of a solution. Westsal, for example, contained lithium chloride, citric acid and potassium iodide, all dissolved in water.[8] The patient sprinkled the solution on to his food to obtain the salty flavour. Of course, the dose of lithium which was administered in this way was completely uncontrolled and it was perhaps not surprising that reports of toxic reactions began to appear.

In February 1949, a number of newspapers in the USA carried warnings about the likely harmful effects of lithium-containing salt substitutes, and local and national radio stations reinforced this with broadcast messages to the same effect. On the last day of that month, *Time* magazine published a brief report[9] headed 'Case of the substitute salt' which is worth quoting here in full:

> People with high blood pressure, or some diseases of the heart and kidneys, are often forbidden to use salt. Last spring the Foster-Milburn Co. of Buffalo thought it had found something harmless that would give food a salty flavor. The new product, Westsal, contained lithium chloride (table salt is sodium chloride).
>
> Early this month, doctors at a Manhattan hospital suspected that the substitute salt might have played a part in the death of a patient with heart disease. The Food & Drug Administration began experimenting and found that heavy doses of lithium chloride killed laboratory animals. Then the FDA checked up on human patients taking the salt, and found that they were suffering variously from drowsiness, weakness, loss of appetite, nausea, tremors, blurred vision, unconsciousness.
>
> Whether the symptoms were due to the patients' diseases or to the lithium chloride, no one could positively say – at the time. But to play safe, the FDA ordered the Foster-Milburn Co. and two other manufacturers[10] of similar products to take them off the market.
>
> Last week the case of the strange salt suddenly became more serious. A doctor in Ann Arbor, Mich. reported to Dr Morris Fishbein, editor of the *Journal of the American Medical Association*, that a patient was critically ill, apparently from lithium chloride. Two days later three doctors from Cleveland's Crile Clinic sent in another report: two patients (one 70, the other 60) had died and five others were ill, apparently from the salt. Dr Fishbein asked newspapers and radio stations to issue warnings. Planning to re-classify lithium chloride as a drug instead of as a special dietary food, FDA heard of the deaths and warned: 'Stop using this dangerous poison at once'.[11]

This news item preceded publication of the relevant clinical details in the medical literature. The 'doctors at a Manhattan hospital'[12] were Lawrence Hanlon, Mason Romaine, Frank Gilroy and John Deitrick: their report[13] was printed in the *Journal of the American Medical Association* of 12 March 1949, just under two weeks after the appearance of the article in *Time*. The patient with heart disease, referred to by *Time*, cannot be identified with any certainty from the report of Lawrence Hanlon and his colleagues, since seven cases were described, three of which involved patients with cardiac problems: two of the three patients (both having heart disease) died as a result of lithium toxicity occasioned by Westsal.

The results of the investigation carried out on lithium toxicity by the Food and Drug Administration using animal subjects (rats and dogs), must have been available in 1949 in order for the general conclusions to be quoted by *Time* magazine, but the full report did not appear in print until 1950.[14]

The 'doctor in Ann Arbor'[15] was Dr A. M. Waldron. His letter[16] to the editor of the *Journal of the American Medical Association* was published in the same issue of the journal as contained the longer and more detailed article of Hanlon and his associates.[17] Waldron's comments were, despite the tone of the *Time* article, relatively mild. He noted that in four patients, symptoms such as tremor, disturbed gait, general weakness, exhaustion and blurred vision, which were all traceable to the consumption of Westsal by the patients, disappeared following withdrawal of the salt substitute and did not recur. Waldron did not go as far as recommending that Westsal should not be used, but only that 'the practitioner should be warned of its possible toxic reactions, so that he may be on the lookout for them'.[18] There was no support in anything that Waldron said for the assertion made in *Time* that 'a patient was critically ill, apparently from lithium chloride',[19] though since *Time* published the information before anything appeared in the *Journal of the American Medical Association* it may be that this phrase, or something like it, was used in the verbal communications which passed between Morris Fishbein, editor of the *Journal*, and *Time* magazine's reporter (possibly at Fishbein's instigation since he was clearly concerned with achieving maximum publicity for the toxic effects of lithium).

Nevertheless, that lithium salts were not only toxic but, in sufficient quantity, lethal, was amply shown by the 'three doctors from Cleveland's Crile Clinic',[20] A. C. Corcoran, R. D. Taylor and Irvine Page, who reported[21] two deaths and five cases of severe but reversible toxic reactions in which lithium ingestion, in the form of Westsal, was clearly implicated. Their account of these fatalities appeared in the issue of the *Journal of the American Medical Association* which contained the articles by Waldron and by Hanlon's group, as well as an account by Robert Stern of a patient showing severe lithium toxicity caused by Westsal.[22] Taken together, the four reports sounded a loud and very clear warning against the continued use of lithium-based salt substitutes.

The United States Food and Drugs Administration (FDA) acted quickly. Even in advance of the publication of the toxicity reports it issued a public warning that Westsal, Foodsal and Salti-salt should be regarded as dangerous.[23] The fourth type of salt substitute, Milosal, was not included in the warning since, '. . . when inquiry was first made of Milani Diafood by the Food & Drug Administration, the firm acknowledged that it had been experimenting with the production of a lithium-chloride-containing salt substitute, but stated that there had not been any interstate distribution of the article'.[24] Milosal had, however, not only been distributed but found its way into certain hospitals and sanitaria, and quanities were possessed by salesmen and distributors throughout the USA. Milosal became the subject of a separate FDA warning.[25] Two days after the appearance of the *Time* magazine article, the FDA published a more general warning against the continued use of all available salt substitutes, including those containing no lithium:

> There is considerable doubt as to the safety of unrestricted use of *any* salt substitute in the presence of cardiovascular-renal disease and a low sodium diet .... The interstate distribution of each salt substitute should be discontinued until a new drug application has been filed and has become effective with respect to the substitute.[26]

Despite its efforts, the FDA failed to satisfy its sterner critics. The Medical Adviser to the Health and Medicine of *Consumer Reports*[27] took the FDA severely to task for failing to act before deaths had occurred from lithium poisoning, particularly in view of the evidence obtained from studies carried out on animals in the FDA laboratories.[28]

> Perhaps the FDA is understaffed to handle its all-important work, and just didn't get around to lithium chloride. Perhaps it weighed the evidence of harmfulness against the defense it knew the sellers of lithium chloride would put up (including testimonials from a number of physicians) and decided not to risk a court battle. Whatever the reason, it is clear that the FDA had reason to challenge lithium chloride ... had the power at least to bring charges after the salts were marketed, and failed to do so until tragedy forced its hand.[29]

If all this was true, then what had gone wrong? In the first place, the laws then governing the powers of the FDA made an important distinction between a 'drug' and a 'food'. The controls which the FDA could exercise upon new drugs were considerable, and any drug product being marketed for the first time was required to satisfy a variety of fairly stringent requirements in respect of its composition, methods of manufacture, distribution and marketing. If, however, a product was classified not as a drug but as a foodstuff, the powers of the FDA to control or delay marketing were virtually nil. Only after marketing had taken place could the FDA act, and even then it was the FDA and not the manufacturers upon whom the onus rested to provide the evidence on which a decision to stop or to continue production could be based – a time-consuming and costly procedure. Lithium chloride, since it was included in a taste substitute preparation, or a 'special dietary food', had thus been classified as a food itself and not as a drug: the FDA was then powerless to do more than wait and see.

The question naturally arises as to whether the FDA was ever justified in its original allocation of the lithium salt to the food category. Certainly, such a move might have been defensible had the evidence for its toxic potential been absent, scanty or equivocal. In fact, not only had the FDA obtained clear information from its own laboratory investigations that lithium salts could lead to toxic reactions, but there were abundant indications in the literature that this was the case, both in man and in other animals. The reports, moreover, were not only relatively recent ones: knowledge of untoward effects arising from lithium administration had been available for at least eighty years.

Pre-1949 reports of lithium toxicity

Perhaps the first indication that lithium salts might produce effects which resulted in discomfort or inconvenience to the recipient, came from Alexander Ure who, in 1860, reported[30] that the injection of a solution of lithium carbonate directly into the bladder led to diuresis and nocturnal difficulties in retaining urine. Indeed, the diuretic effects of lithium, indicating a possible lithium-induced disturbance of kidney function, was a recurring theme throughout the early reports on lithium effects.

The next to notice and comment upon this particular property was George Duncan Gibb[31] in 1865; Gibb put forward the suggestion that lithium bromide might be usefully employed as a diuretic, particularly when combined with other substances possessing a similar action.

Lithium-induced diuresis was well known to Garrod who mentioned the fact in his articles in the *Medical Times and Gazette* of 1873,[32] and again in the third edition of his treatise on gout:[32]

> All the salts of lithia appear to be powerful diuretics, in some patients increasing the flow of urine to a somewhat annoying extent; and I have known many instances in which a bottle of lithia water, taken at bedtime, would cause the patient to be disturbed during the night, whereas the same quantity of soda-water would produce no such result.[34]

In one of Garrod's patients, lithium was administered over a seven-year period and the patient remained free from gout and calculi during that time. At the dose levels used, Garrod occasionally observed a fine tremor in the hands and arms (a symptom now well known as a virtually ubiquitous side effect of lithium treatment) and he commented that he had been informed of similar symptoms having been noted by others – thereby clearly indicating that his remedy for gout must have been taken up by other physicians shortly after the appearance of the first edition of his book in 1859[35] and that the occurrence of lithium-induced side effects had become a matter of fairly common knowledge. Garrod kept careful note of untoward effects produced by lithium, and the third edition of his book in 1876[36] carried an interesting list:

In two cases I have noticed a slight trembling of one hand produced by their [lithium salts] use; in both patients there existed some kidney mischief; and in a third case slight twitching of both arms occurred when the patient was taking very large doses. I have also heard of the case of a gentleman who thought it produced some not well-defined nervous symptoms; the patient notwithstanding continued the medicine, as it gave relief to his gout. Dr Charcot states, in his annotations to the French edition of this work, that he has given carbonate of lithia to the extent of 39 and 45 grains in the 24 hours without the production of any unpleasant symptoms. In larger doses continued for some days, dyspepsia was often produced.[37]

It was, in all probability, Garrod's publicising of the diuretic action of lithium, rather than the very brief and obscure report published by Gibb, which led to the clinical use of lithium salts as diuretics. A number of subsequent authors, in commenting upon this property, referred to Garrod's book[38] as their authority.

The earliest study of more general toxicological properties of lithium seems to have been that of Rambuteau in 1868[39] who reported vomiting and diarrhoea in a dog given 20 grains of the sulphate.

Five years later, in 1873, James Blake[40] noted that 1 grain of lithium sulphate per kilo bodyweight was a lethal dose in rabbits.

Hesse, in 1876,[41] gave a more detailed description of lithium-induced physiological changes, mentioning reduced neural excitability, lowered body temperature and diuresis as particular responses observed in rabbits. The same kind of neural effect was observed in frogs by Brunton and Cash in 1884,[42] whilst Krumhoff[43] in the same year, found cardiovascular side effects, vomiting, diarrhoea, and ultimately death, to result from intravenous, subcutaneous and oral administration of lithium chloride to animals. Charles Richet, in 1886,[44] reported that 0.1 g of lithium chloride injected into a rabbit led to the animal's death after two or three days: the fatal outcome was preceded by a gradual drop in body temperature, effects upon the heart and digestion, and a fall in bodyweight. In dogs, nervous system functioning was disrupted and an intense diarrhoea was noted. Subcutaneous injection of 0.23 g of lithium chloride led to the dogs' death in one and a half hours. Similar effects were observed in pigeons, guinea-pigs, fish, frogs and crayfish. In 1892, a Swiss pharmacologist, Paul Binet[45] recorded that lithium was very toxic in frogs, and was indeed the most toxic of all the alkali and alkaline earth metals.

Whilst these toxicological investigations produced quite alarming results, scant regard was paid to the findings by those using lithium salts therapeutically towards the end of the nineteenth century.

Lithium intoxication first started to become a matter of concern with the general availablity of tablets for producing lithia water.[46] Since this enabled a large number of people to self-administer fairly large and uncontrolled quantities of lithium, it was inevitable that a number of cases of lithium intoxication should arise – many more, in all probability, than were ever recognised as such, and certainly considerably more than were recorded in the literature. In 1898, Dr Louis Kolipinski read a paper before the Therapeutic Society of the District of Columbia,[47] in which he described two patients suffering from conditions which could be traced directly to lithium poisoning resulting from drinking lithia water prepared from tablets. Amongst the symptoms were fine tremor and a general impairment of muscular competence, the same effects that Garrod had described and which were later to become so well known to those prescribing lithium treatment.

With the coming of the twentieth century, knowledge increased about the toxic properties of lithium salts, and there occurred a growing awareness on the part of the medical profession that the therapeutic use of lithium was not without its attendant dangers. To large measure this was due to the detailed toxicological studies on cats carried out by Clarence Good at the University of Michigan and published in the widely read and influential *American Journal of Medical Science* in 1903.[48] A number of physicians, influenced by this report, warned against the unrestricted use of lithium salts for conditions such as gout. For example, Dr Arthur Luff, writing in 1907 on the treatment of gout,[49] made the point very forcefully:

> As regards the use of lithium salts in the treatment of gout, my opinion is that they are not so useful as the potassium and sodium salts. The principal objection to their use is their greater toxicity, and depressing action on the heart, as compared with the potassium salts. . . . I constantly meet with patients suffering from cardiac depression, and even dilatation, as the result of the excessive and continued consumption of lithia tablets.[50]

The first description of subjective effects resulting from lithium intoxication was provided by Dr S. A. Cleaveland[51] of Western Reserve University, ten years after the publication of Good's report. Cleaveland's account of his attempt to poison himself with what he called, rather curiously, lithium 'chlorid', makes interesting reading and is reproduced here in full:

> During an investigation on the action of uric acid under Professor Haskins, I had occasion to take rather large doses of lithium chlorid, and experienced toxic symptoms differing in some respects from the hitherto described phenomena of lithium poisoning.
>
> In the first experiment, 2 gm. of the chlorid were taken in a glass of water after each meal for three meals (about 1 p.m., 9 p.m. and 7 a.m.) and then, after skipping one meal, another dose was taken about 7 p.m., making a total of 8 gm., about 125 grains, in twenty-eight hours. Symptoms showed themselves three or four hours after the first dose, consisting in slight dizziness and fulness in the head. Nothing more was noted after

the second dose, which was taken in the evening. Soon after the third dose there was so much blurring of vision that it was impossible to read anything smaller than the largest headlines of a newspaper.

Dizziness and ringing in the ears were quite marked. There were also great general weakness and marked tremors. The fourth dose was taken at night, and the dizziness became so marked that the room seemed to go round all night, and sleep was almost impossible. The next morning the condition approached prostration. The eye symptoms were exaggerated and the dizziness, weakness and tremors were so intense that there was staggering and it was necessary to go to bed. The eye and ear symptoms lasted about a day and a half after the last dose. The weakness and tremors persisted for five days. At no time were there any gastro-intestinal symptoms – there was no abdominal pain, diarrhea or gastric irritation, and the appetite was very good throughout the whole time.

Several months later the experiment was repeated to make certain that the effects were really due to lithium. Only two doses of 2 gm. each were necessary to bring on the dizziness, ringing in the ears and blurring of vision. The general symptoms were much less marked than before, but there was some weakness for a day or so. Again there were no gastro-intestinal effects.

The notable features of these observations are the marked muscular and general prostration; the occurrence of vertigo and eye and ear symptoms resembling those of cinchonism, and the entire absence of gastro-intestinal symptoms.

According to literature of lithium poisoning, as quoted by Good,[52] the common symptoms consist in marked prostration and gastro-intestinal irritation. The latter was entirely absent in my case, while the striking cinchonism effects do not appear to have been described by any previous reporters; but the doses taken by me (60 to 90 grains per day) were two or three times greater than those which seem to have been taken in the cases reported in the literature.[53]

After Cleaveland's report, relatively little[54] appeared in the literature concerning lithium side effects and toxicity until 1949; nevertheless, there is clearly considerable justice in the claim made in *Consumer Reports* for 1949[55] to the effect that information about lithium toxicity had been readily available for a long time and could therefore have been used by the FDA to prevent or delay the sale of lithium-containing salt substitutes.

Aftermath of the salt substitute debacle

So much publicity was given to the toxic properties of the salt substitutes that it stimulated a number of further reports of a similar nature. Dr Henry Peters of Madison, Wisconsin[56] gave an account of a reversible choreoathetotic state due to Westsal, and Irwin Greenfield with a group of his colleagues from the Kings County Hospital, New York,[57] presented case reports of two further patients, both of whom showed lithium toxicity after using Westsal. Several toxicological investigations using animal subjects followed rapidly[58] and generally confirmed that lithium salts could produce marked effects on a number of important physiological systems.

When John Cade started using lithium salts to control manic excitement he was apparently quite unaware of the deaths and toxic reactions being caused by lithium contained in salt substitutes. No comparable substances were produced or marketed outside the USA and the panic which was stirred up by the *Journal of the American Medical Association* and by the pronouncements of the FDA, went almost unremarked by the rest of the world. It was not long, however, before a fatality occurred in a patient receiving lithium treatment for mania and, in August 1950, Dr E. L. Roberts published a brief report in the *Medical Journal of Australia*[59] describing just such a case. The connection was immediately established between lithium salts used as salt substitutes and as therapeutic agents in psychiatry, and it is hardly surprising that clinicians who might otherwise have welcomed an apparently effective, and possibly specific, antimanic medication, were reluctant to expose their patients to the risk of harmful side effects.

Not that lithium was without its defenders, however. Dr J. V. Ashburner, Senior Medical Officer at the Sunbury Mental Hospital, Victoria, was quick to try to counter the impression given by Roberts. In a letter to the editor of the *Medical Journal of Australia*,[60] Ashburner wrote about his experiences with lithium treatment in more than fifty patients and recorded that in his hospital thirteen pounds of lithium carbonate and two pounds of citrate had been consumed by patients since the publication of Cade's article just over a year previously. Whilst agreeing that 'minor toxic manifestations are not uncommon',[61] Ashburner claimed that none was irreversible following dosage reduction. He expressed the hope that Roberts' report would not create an unfavourable impression about lithium.

A strong defence of lithium-containing salt substitutes was made at about the same time by John Talbott.[62] Talbott's interest in lithium had arisen partly from his work on gout and uric acid, and partly from investigations he had carried out on acid–base balance in certain metabolic disorders, in which studies low sodium chloride diets had been used. His studies on gout and uric acid caused him to conclude that lithium salts were ineffective in increasing uric acid secretion and were thus not useful in the treatment of gout; his search for a salt substitute for his patients in the metabolic disorder experiments had led him to ammonium and potassium salts but not lithium salts. These two facets of his previous experience were brought together in 1949 when he was asked to investigate the acceptability of a new salt substitute which consisted of a solution of lithium chloride and citric acid in water, with a trace of potassium iodide.[63] Talbott's report of the outcome of this work appeared in 1950, after the storm had broken over lithium toxicity.

He noted that in only three cases out of more than fifty investigated had any symptoms appeared showing any similarity to those described in the reports of toxicity. Even when much larger doses[64] were used the only untoward effect was described as 'some gastro-intestinal distress'.[65] Talbott extended his studies to rats, pro-rating the lithium chloride for bodyweight so as to give the rats the equivalent of about seven times the human average daily intake: again he found little evidence of toxic effects even though the lithium administration extended over eight weeks. Eventually, field trials were done 'in the eastern portion of the country',[66] and when there was no report of unwanted reactions, the salt substitute was made generally available.

Talbott was probably the first person to monitor serum lithium levels and to correlate them with the occurrence of side effects and toxic reactions, and this was a particularly important element in the defence which he tried to make for the salt substitutes. Talbott's description of the lithium toxicity panic and of the steps which he himself took in an attempt to bring a little objectivity to the situation is worth quoting at some length:

Near the conclusion of these studies, I was notified that a death alleged to be associated with excessive lithium intake had been reported to the manufacturers [of the salt substitute]. I also learned that after a conference with the Federal Food and Drug Administration all lithium substitutes for salt had been withdrawn from the market and steps had been taken to recall outstanding stocks. One manufacturer immediately mailed a letter to all physicians notifying them of this step and of the reported possibility of untoward effects. Ten days after the withdrawal from the market the report of several deaths, alleged to have been caused by lithium poisoning, was broadcast. No advance notice of this broadcast, in order that physicians could prepare the several thousands of patients taking these salt substitutes for the alarming statements, was given the physicians, druggists or manufacturers by those responsible for the dissemination of the report. The prescribing physician was embarrassed in many instances by a deluge of telephone calls from his patients requesting advice, and the only information available was that reported over the air and in the newspapers. It is believed that the situation was not so serious as one was led to believe from the lay reports.

During the following days, a great number of physicians sought additional information, many times to obtain guidance in discussing the situation with patients and a few times to report cases of possible poisoning. In each instance of the latter situation a request was made to the attending physician for a sample of blood for determination of the lithium level in the serum. Blood from 9 patients was submitted for analysis. . . . In only 2 instances was the concentration of lithium greater than 0.7 milliequivalents; these values were 1.4 and 1.9 milliequivalents, respectively. . . . In the study of normal subjects untoward symptoms were observed only when the serum lithium was above 0.7 milliequivalents.

Moreover, in the hospital patients I observed serum lithium concentrations as high as 2.9 milliequivalents without the appearence of untoward effects, and except in 1 case I did not observe signs of intoxication until serum lithium levels reached 2.3 milliequivalents.[67]

Moreover, in the case of 2 of the 3 patients who showed the highest serum lithium levels it was noted that a low serum sodium level was also present. The patient with a serum lithium concentration of 1.4 milliequivalents had a serum sodium level of 119.0 milliequivalents, and the one with a serum lithium concentration of 0.7 milliequivalents had a serum sodium level of 132.0 milliequivalents; yet, a third patient with a serum lithium concentration of 1.9 milliequivalents had a serum sodium level of 137.0 milliequivalents.

The incidence of valid reactions due to the ingestion of lithium is unknown. Following the indiscriminate press and radio publicity an attempt was made in this clinic and others to contact hundreds of lithium users in order to obtain more precise information. The alarm had so frightened the majority of those who used the substitute that many symptoms, regardless of cause, were attributed to the ingestion of lithium. I myself have seen several patients claiming lithium intoxication whose symptoms, on close inquiry, were found to be due to other causes.[68]

Talbott then turned his attention to the various published reports of lithium toxicity and pointed out that, in nearly all the cases described, the average daily intake of lithium chloride was greatly in excess of that found to be safe in his own patients. Moreover, he argued that 'many of the individual symptoms that have been attributed to lithium intoxication may in a cardiac or hypertensive patient appear quite independently of the intake of lithium', and added that 'several of these symptoms may be induced in normal persons on a rigidly low sodium intake'.[69] There was, indeed, quite independent support for this latter proposition. In 1949, the year of Cade's discovery and one year before Talbott's paper, the *Journal of the American Medical Association* had carried a detailed report by Louis Soloff and Jacob Zatuchni[70] in which the syndrome of salt depletion was graphically outlined: these authors noted that 'no salt substitute was used by any of these patients, so that neither lithium nor potassium intoxication had to be considered as possible aggravating factors'.[71] Death from sodium depletion was clearly a sufficient explanation for many of the cases which had been ascribed to lithium intoxication.

Talbott's paper was, seen in retrospect, one of the most important contributions to the founding of modern lithium therapy: it established the practice of routine serum lithium monitoring to avoid intoxication and it made quite explicit the importance of an adequate intake of sodium.[72] It failed, however, to reverse completely the damage that had been done to the reputation of lithium, and the next few years saw lithium therapy used only sporadically.

5

Early confirmations

A cautious beginning

John Cade's report of lithium treatment of mania might well have suc-
cumbed to the same fate as that suffered by many proposed therapeutic
techniques both before and after that time – an initial interest being followed
by dismissal as soon as adverse effects were shown or suspected to occur.
Had lithium salts been at all expensive or hard to come by, it is doubtful
whether their therapeutic applications in psychiatry would ever have been
investigated any further. Thanks, however, to the persistence into the
mid-twentieth century of the uric acid diathesis,[1] canisters of lithium salts
(usually as effervescent preparations) were to be found in most hospital
pharmacies. It was thus a relatively simple matter for any psychiatrist, whose
interest had been stirred by Cade's article, to try for himself the effects of
lithium on manic or hypomanic patients. This probably happened in more
hospitals than ever reported the fact, particularly since the toxicity scare may
have led to lithium rapidly being withdrawn from some patients as psychiatrists hurried to protect themselves against a charge of administering a
harmful substance.

One particularly interesting account of an early use of lithium salts has
been given by Dr R. M. Young[2] who, in 1949, was Deputy Medical
Superintendent of Parkside Hospital at Macclesfield, England. Dr Young
was certainly one of the first in England to use lithium salts as the treatment
of choice in mania.

> I saw a summary of the original article in the *Australian Medical Journal*
> of 1948 or '49[3] ... in the abstracts prepared for the 'Institute of Living',
> Hertford, Conn., and found a supply of effervescent lithium citrate on a
> back shelf of the Dispensary of Parkside Hospital ... I think this prepara-
> tion had been recommended in the past as a health-giving mineral water[4]
> but had not had much popularity. As instructed in the Australian article, I

gave the citrate in double the dose by weight recommended for the carbonate and was immediately converted by the dramatic way in which the manic symptoms were switched off in a few days in cases particularly of mild hypomania who were such a disruptive influence in a quiet ward. The treatment of choice in acute mania and acute delirious mania was well modified ECT, but not infrequently a chronic hypomania supervened which was almost more difficult to cope with before lithium proved to be the answer.

I soon realised that lithium was dangerous in cases where exhaustion or dehydration was present as a result of the more acute manic states, and made a practice of using ECT first in such cases. Dosage was, I think, 30 grains of the citrate or 15 of the carbonate three times a day until the mania switched off, and then once daily indefinitely.

There was no information about supervising blood levels and my half-hearted attempts to interest the pathologists in research failed, as I think they thought I was a mad psychiatrist playing with dangerous chemicals.

I soon found that lithium seemed if anything, harmful in endogenous depressive states and the depressive phase of manic depressive episodes, and though I used lithium to prevent recurrences in purely manic cases, unfortunately I never used it between attacks to prevent depressive relapses, as has become regular practice since my retirement.

The occurrence of several near disasters made me turn to phenothiazines when they appeared, but I never felt they were specific, and I continued to use lithium off and on when I felt it indicated. . . .

Unfortunately pressure of work, expanding services in the community in the Manchester Region ... prevented my publishing, though I spread the word by word of mouth to my colleagues in the early 'fifties. They also however were tempted by the more respectable and, to the drug firms, more profitable, phenothiazines, so I was rather a lone voice preaching in competition with mass advertising. I gather the salts of lithium cost almost nothing to produce.

In a letter to the editor of the *Medical Journal of Australia*,[5] Dr J. V. (Val) Ashburner referred, in 1950, to a large number of cases of mania successfully treated with lithium in his hospital. This was the first published account of the antimanic potential of lithium since Cade's own report had appeared in the same journal the previous year,[6] but it gave few precise details.

Ashburner has subsequently explained how it was that he came to use lithium.[7]

I was from 1947 to 1950 Senior Medical Officer at Sunbury Mental Hospital, recently discharged from the Australian Army, where I had been Director of Psychology 1942–46. I was, therefore, seized with interest in being up-to-date in experimental method and in what is now called cost–benefit. The situation at Sunbury, an old asylum run down by the war conditions, was dreadful. I had virtually no facilities. . . .

At a meeting of perhaps a dozen of my colleagues at Royal Park called to discuss clinical matters, Cade produced, and read briefly, his forthcoming paper, which was to be the first paper on lithium treatment. We discussed the matter fully. With the brashness that went in all medicine at that time, most of us went home to our hospitals to see if we could find out more about this promising stuff. I went to the pharmacist at Sunbury Mental Hospital and asked him if we had any lithium chloride or lithium citrate in stock, since these were the only substances that Cade mentioned in discussion of his paper. The pharmacist replied 'no, but I have a bloody big jar of carbonate'. This, I think, was a relic of some decades earlier when there was a vogue for using lithium for the treatment of rheumatism. We concocted a suspension of lithium carbonate with tragacanth, flavoured with tincture of ginger, and made up to half ounce doses, each containing 10 grains of lithium carbonate. This, for me, was the start of lithium treatment. I looked round to see who may possibly be helped. My philosophy then, with anything new, was to be sceptical of a one-to-one relationship between diagnosis and so-called remedy. I therefore gave lithium carbonate to a select group of patients who had one thing in common – excitation – but were not all manic. Some I can recall vividly. . . . Like myself, the other psychiatrists were working alone except for the small group centered round Cade in the Mont Park area; but we communicated freely. . . . I did know Cade was having trouble with toxicity, but I was able to contrast all his difficulties with my singular lack of problems. He was using the chloride and citrate and did not change over to carbonate only, until somewhat later. The soluble salts were much more dangerous than the carbonate, having a narrower safe therapeutic dose range. . . .

There was no opposition to the use of lithium. In those days people tended to assume that doctors knew what they were doing, and my colleagues either used it themselves or were asylum doctors who didn't use anything. . . . I was just amongst the few clinicians who were in the right place at the right time, and in no sense was I working 'with' Cade or the group mentioned above. My activities within the hospital were chiefly concerned with its social structure, and the modification of this so as to develop group patterns of change.

The work of E. M. Trautner

Also in Australia, and at about the same time as Ashburner was trying out lithium salts, two investigators in the Department of Physiology of the University of Melbourne, C. H. Noack and E. M. Trautner,[8] decided to make a detailed study of both toxicity and therapeutic response resulting from lithium administration.

It so happened that the intellectual climate in Melbourne was exactly right for Noack and Trautner's work to prosper, and this was in large measure due to a young Research Fellow, Dr Victor Wynn.[9] Wynn had been a medical officer in the Royal Australian Army and during his service had seen cases of renal failure resulting from potassium poisoning; in order to investigate the general issue of water and electrolyte balance, Wynn joined the Department of Physiology at Melbourne University in 1948 in an unpaid capacity.[10] He realised that the available methods for quantitative estimation of potassium levels in biological tissues were both cumbersome and inaccurate and he sought a new technique: this he found in the flame spectrophotometer, of which at that time only three or four were in use anywhere in the world (for agricultural work such as soil analysis). Wynn approached the Beckmann Instrument Company in the USA who manufactured the flame spectrophotometer and persuaded them to release one of the two which they had available, the purchase being made by Wynn himself with funds which he personally raised. The Beckman Company were intrigued by Wynn's proposal to use the flame spectrophotometer in clinical work, but Wynn replied that in his view the potential of the apparatus was such that within a very few years there would be one in every major clinical medical unit in the world. Heading a small team of five investigators, under the auspices of the then Professor of Physiology at Melbourne, R. Douglas Wright, Wynn set out to apply the new technique of flame spectrophotometry to sodium and potassium analyses in biological fluids, and in 1950 the group published an account of the first ever use of the instrument in clinical chemistry.[11] Trautner thus found himself in an environment in which notions of ionic regulation were being actively discussed, and in which the means for studying quantitative aspects of electrolytes were readily available. When Cade's report appeared concerning the effects of lithium on manic psychosis, Trautner persuaded C. H. Noack (a member of the class to which Trautner gave instruction for the Diploma of Psychological Medicine) to follow up the question of safe lithium levels and signs of intoxication. Trautner approached Victor Wynn and asked him whether he could run some serum samples through his flame spectrophotometer in order to assess lithium levels. Wynn readily agreed and made the point to Trautner that, in view of the chemical similarities between lithium and potassium, it was more than likely that close supervision of serum lithium levels would be necessary to avoid the kind of toxic effects which Wynn knew to be produced by excess potassium. Noack and Trautner took this advice and carefully monitored all their clinical cases.[12] Their findings, based on work with more than a hundred patients were published in August 1951, in the *Medical Journal of Australia*[13] as an article which, in its own way, was probably as influential as Cade's original report in promoting lithium therapy. Not only did Noack and Trautner confirm Cade's observation that lithium was an effective antimanic agent, but they addressed themselves directly to the question uppermost in the minds of those psychiatrists contemplating trying lithium treatment, namely whether or not the toxic reactions and side effects resulting from the use of lithium were sufficiently marked and serious to offset any therapeutic advantages which the treatment might possess. Their conclusion was optimistic:

> We did not meet with any serious cases of intoxication among over 100 patients suffering from different mental diseases. In view of the very beneficial effect of the drug in the cases of mania reported, it does not appear to be justified to abandon lithium as a form of medication solely because some fatal cases have been reported in which lithium poisoning has been incriminated; it appears rather that attempts should be made to establish clinical criteria which will result in a better selection of suitable cases.[14]

In his defence of lithium-based salt substitutes, John Talbott[15] had introduced the use of serum lithium measurements as a means of indexing the toxic levels of lithium. This technique was adopted by Noack and Trautner to great effect. They established a set of basic guidelines for establishing and monitoring safe serum lithium levels, which were subsequently to be the cornerstone of further developments in the practical management of lithium therapy: it is, indeed, difficult to overemphasise the importance of the contribution which Noack and Trautner's article eventually made to the re-establishment of lithium therapy as a viable and acceptable proposition in psychiatry following the bad press which had stemmed from the toxicity panic of 1949,[16] though its immediate impact was, as will be seen later,[17] probably not very great.

Whilst Cade's findings produced their greatest initial impact in Australia (perhaps understandably), a number of reports soon began to appear of clinical studies carried out in European centres, particularly in France. It is by no means clear why the French should have been so interested in lithium therapy, unless the fact that mineral springs were (and still are) so popular in that country predisposed the clinicians to respond positively to any suggestion that a naturally-occurring substance (and one, moreover, reputed to be present in certain spring waters) might possess therapeutic properties. Whatever the reason, between 1951 and 1955 there were ten clinical reports from France,[18] as against one from Italy,[19] four from Australia,[20] and two from Denmark.[21] The French reports all carried more or less the same message: lithium therapy, administered in accordance with Cade's prescription, seemed to be fairly effective against most cases of psycho-motor excitation, but particularly so against the excitation of mania:

> On peut simplement remarquer que l'action semble plus nette dans la manie que dans les autres états d'excitation.[22]

Whilst only fairly mild side effects were noted, the treatment being in general found to be relatively free from such complications, Drs N. Duc and

H. Maurel,[23] from Montpellier, did make special reference to the closeness of therapeutic and toxic dose levels. In not one French study, however, were serum lithium levels determined in the course of treatment; nor were they in the single reported Italian investigation.[24] It may be that this was one of the main reasons for these reports failing to have much impact on psychiatric practice, since although they reaffirmed the therapeutic effectiveness of lithium, they provided the potential prescriber with no assurance that the treatment would not prove harmful, and they did not suggest ways and means by which treatment could be monitored so as to reduce to a minimum the risks of toxic reactions occurring or, having occurred, progressing. If general acceptance of lithium therapy were to be secured in the aftermath of the alarm generated by the toxicity scare, it was clearly going to be necessary to establish very clear guidelines for its safe administration, particularly since reports continued to appear sporadically in the literature dealing with cases of lithium intoxication, occasionally of a serious nature.[25]

In Australia, Trautner and his group continued to explore the way in which ingested lithium was retained by and excreted from the body, and in 1955 a detailed account of their findings was published in the *Medical Journal of Australia*.[26] Whilst the primary stated aim of the work was to determine lithium effects on ionic balance, the article actually provided all that was needed for the development of a rational and safe lithium administration procedure and there can be no doubt that, because of this, the work helped to some extent to maintain interest in lithium therapy. Opinions differ, however, as to the weight which should be assigned to Trautner's role at this stage in the development of lithium therapy. Dr Samuel Gershon, one-time colleague of Trautner[27] has no doubt that Trautner had a major influence:

It was Dr Trautner who first used plasma lithium assays in his studies. Altogether Dr Trautner's exceedingly important role in the early studies on lithium has sadly been completely neglected.[28]

Professor R. Douglas Wright echoes the sentiment:

I . . . believe that his part in the lithium story has been overshadowed.[29]

Dr J. V. Ashburner, however, thinks otherwise:

From the point of view of the practising clinician away from the university scene, his work meant practically nothing.[30]

In a sense, both evaluations are probably correct. There were those who, like Sam Gershon, were convinced by Trautner's work that lithium treatment could be both effective and safe, and who proceeded subsequently to act upon their conviction by undertaking lithium therapy with plasma monitoring as an integral part of the procedure. Gershon was later to go to the USA where he played a leading role in establishing lithium therapy in that country.[31] On the other hand, Val Ashburner's assessment of Trautner's work as not particularly meaningful to the clinician, whilst perhaps being a rather harsh judgement, is not without substance: Trautner was not himself a clinician, his primary interest in lithium being biochemical, and the whole tenor of his published work reflects this orientation. In his major report on lithium excretion and retention,[32] he used normal volunteers as well as patients, specifically disclaiming a major concern with the therapeutic aspects of his work:

> Clinical observations are reported, in so far as they seem to modify the interpretation of the results obtained in the healthy, or to indicate promising lines of more detailed investigation. No extensive clinical discussion is intended.[33]

This may well have caused many psychiatrists either to overlook Trautner's work or to regard it as too theoretical to be of direct concern to the practicalities of treatment.

The work of B. Glesinger

In 1954 the *Medical Journal of Australia* carried a long and detailed evaluation of lithium treatment, written by Dr B. Glesinger, a psychiatrist at Claremont Mental Hospital, Western Australia.[34] This was, in many ways, a remarkable piece of writing. Glesinger had researched his subject thoroughly. He carefully detailed the results of his own findings, indicating which diagnostic groups had responded well, and which poorly, to lithium treatment. Side effects were described in great detail and the review of the literature on lithium toxicity was thorough and painstaking. There can be no doubt but that Glesinger's article will have provided a solid foundation upon which others who might be interested in investigating lithium could build. There are some curious remarks made about patient management.

> There is no necessity to measure or control lithium excretion by complicated chemical methods or to determine the plasma content. This refinement can be reserved for institutions with appropriate facilities. Lithium treatment can be carried out in any hospital safely and even at home under supervision.[35]

In other respects, however, Glesinger's recommendations on patient management were excellent and his positive conclusion that lithium 'represents a step forward towards the ideal treatment ... is easy and safe to administer, and ... is usable for a fairly long period'[36] must have encouraged many psychiatrists to look carefully at the possibility of using lithium treatment in their own institutions.

What was needed to get lithium therapy really moving was a study which presented a clear demonstration of the therapeutic benefits to be obtained by using lithium, together with an unequivocal demonstration that the treatment procedures could be perfectly safe. Such a study was carried out in Denmark and published in *Neurology, Neurosurgery and Psychiatry* in 1954,[37] and it was to prove a major turning point, not only in the fortunes of lithium therapy, but in twentieth-century psychiatry as a whole: it heralded, in fact, the second era of lithium in medicine.

6

Beginning of the second era in medicine

The Danish renaissance of lithium therapy

In 1953, a young Danish psychiatrist by the name of Mogens Schou joined the Department of Psychiatry at Aarhus University Psychiatric Hospital, where he took up the post of research associate with biological psychiatry as his special field.[1] The Head of the Psychiatry Department at that time was Professor Erik Strömgren, and it was he who suggested to Schou that it might make an interesting research topic to investigate further the claims originating from Australia for an antimanic effect of lithium. In Schou's words:

> Equipped with a small laboratory I was looking for appropriate study subjects when Professor Erik Strömgren drew my attention to the Australian reports about lithium treatment of mania.[2]

It was in Denmark that lithium salts had been used by the Lange brothers in the nineteenth century to treat mood disorders,[3] and the question arises as to whether Strömgren's suggestion had its origin in an awareness of this earlier work. Questioned about the matter, Strömgren is doubtful that there was in fact any direct link between the Carl and Frederik Lange reports and his own decision to follow up Cade's findings:

> It is true that the brothers Carl and Frederik (Fritz) Lange used lithium salts in the treatment of mental disorder. Although I knew this I doubt whether it had any influence on the interest I took in the reintroduction of lithium in psychiatric therapy by Cade. But of course . . . knowledge of the old Danish lithium treatment may have prepared me unconsciously and made me sensitive to any new information concerning lithium. To the

conscious parts of my mind, however, it looks as if I was convinced by the first report from Australia that here was really a thing to be taken seriously. In addition I found it extremely fascinating if lithium salts which are chemically so simple could have a therapeutic effect in psychiatry, especially so if they were active against just one disease, which could tell us much more about that disease than lots of information concerning the therapeutic effects of complicated compounds which had no clear preference with regard to the different disorders they were used for. This was the reason why I asked my brilliant younger colleague Mogens Schou to devote himself to lithium studies.[4]

There existed, however, a further link with the Lange brothers: Mogens Schou's father, himself a psychiatrist, had certainly been well acquainted with their work, though he was also very critical of it.[5] Was Mogens Schou aware of this? If so, had he talked to his father about it? Did he know that lithium had already been used in psychiatric practice in Denmark more than fifty years previously? Like Strömgren, Schou denies a connection with the Langes:

Their work played no role for my decision to go into a study of lithium. I cannot remember whether I thought of them at the time, probably not, but I met their work later when I collected material for my large review paper in *Pharmacological Reviews* 1957.[6] The two-and-a-half lines I gave the work there ... indicate the significance, or rather lack of significance, I attach to this work. Their reports were speculative and without any evidence that the treatment worked....

I actually never discussed lithium with my father, because he died in the spring of 1952, before we ever gave lithium to any patient. This does not mean, however, that my father did not play a considerable role for my interest in lithium. He took a life-long interest in biological research concerning manic–depressive disorder and his devotion to this matter certainly influenced me when I decided to become a psychiatrist and to take a particular interest in affective illness.[7]

Indeed, Schou asserts that there were no forces acting to influence his decision to follow up the Australian work other than Strömgren's suggestion. Even the mineral spring connection[8] is summarily dismissed:

I may perhaps at this point add that I also attach little importance to the much quoted observation[9] that various lithium-containing spa waters were used in antiquity. No effect was ever demonstrated by such waters, and I consider it entirely coincidental that they contained lithium (as some of them contained radioactivity and lots of other things). I remember once lecturing in Göttingen, Germany, and during an after-dinner speech I quoted two Göttingen studies on lithium from the late nineteenth century. I think that after-dinner speeches are where these curios belong.[10]

With the collaboration of Professor Strömgren and Drs N. Juel-Nielsen and H. Voldby (psychiatrists who worked in the same hospital) Schou set up a clinical trial to test the claim that lithium had an antimanic therapeutic effect. To thirty-eight manic patients, lithium salts (the citrate, carbonate or chloride) were administered on either an open or double-blind, placebo-controlled basis. According to Schou, this was 'the first or one of the first double-blind trials in psychiatric pharmacotherapy':[11] the findings were published in 1954.[12]

The 1954 report was notable for a number of things. In the first place it broadly verified Cade's original findings, lithium treatment having apparent beneficial effects against mania in a high proportion of cases, and a switch from lithium to placebo having clinical consequences which were generally in the predicted direction.

Secondly, a flame spectrophotometer was used routinely throughout therapy to determine serum sodium, potassium and lithium concentrations, following the practice of Noack and Trautner[13] whose work was referred to several times in the report. It was, in fact, the report by Noack and Trautner which had first alerted Strömgren to lithium, though a copy of Cade's article was quickly obtained. The Noack and Trautner report, being much more detailed than that by Cade, was the more effective promulgator of the idea of lithium treatment, and Schou engaged in correspondence with Trautner on the subject of serum lithium estimations.

Thirdly, close attention was paid to the patterns of toxic reactions and side effects which were observed, and a detailed description of these phenomena, based upon a wide range of laboratory tests, was provided. One patient actually died in the course of therapy, but Schou and his colleagues were disinclined to believe that lithium intoxication was to blame:[14]

The serum lithium level varied usually between 0.5 and 2.0 meq/l during treatment. A serum lithium concentration of 4.5 meq/l was observed in one patient ... who died from an anaemic infarction in the pons (verified by necropsy) after nine days of lithium administration. She was 71 years old, strongly arteriosclerotic, and had had one previous vascular attack during a manic explosion. Lithium treatment was instituted in the hope of preventing her frequent violent manic outbursts. We consider it very unlikely that the lithium medication was responsible for the occurrence of the infarction but rather think that the high serum lithium level may have been caused by a sudden impairment of the patient's general biological functions.[15]

The conclusions drawn were cautious: lithium therapy might be of therapeutic value in some cases of mania, but it was also a potentially dangerous treatment and one which, if undertaken, would require very careful monitoring, both clinically and biochemically.

Over the next few years Schou's group continued to collect data on lithium treatment. By 1955, Schou was able to report that, of forty-eight manic patients treated with lithium alone, thirty-nine (81 per cent) had shown significant clinical improvement.[16] Four years later, in 1959,[17] he was able to add a further 119 patients to this total, of whom ninety-one (76 per cent) had improved under lithium therapy.

In a few other centres similar results were being obtained. From France, two reports[18] referred to a total of thirty-five lithium-treated patients, with an improvement rate of 86 per cent. Samuel Gershon and Edward Trautner[19] in Australia, continuing the work reported five years previously,[20] gave details of a further ten cases (90 per cent improvement). Rice, in what was probably the first report of lithium treatment for mania to come out of England,[21] described thirty-seven cases (92 per cent improvement). In addition there were fourteen cases reported from Italy[22] (93 per cent improvement) and thirty-two from Denmark[23] (75 per cent improvement). In all, since Cade's first report, and including Cade's own figures, Schou's 'stock-taking' as he described it, ten years later, showed a grand total of 370 manic patients[24] treated by lithium alone, of whom 304 (82 per cent) had responded with discernible clinical improvement. To these figures may be added a further 348 from various sources[25] not referred to by Schou; of these, 159 (46 per cent) responded well. The combined improvement rate, taking into account these latter results, was 64 per cent which, though somewhat less than the value presented by Schou,[26] is nevertheless quite impressive for a drug which, only ten years previously, had been branded a dangerous substance.

Having thus decided that there was at least a *prima facie* case for believing lithium to possess an antimanic therapeutic potential, Schou and his associates began to consider the direction which their future researches should take. Schou[27] has stated the problem clearly:

At this point our unit was faced with a choice. Should we attempt gaining insight into the biochemical mode of action of lithium? Or should we concentrate on clinically more relevant topics, therapeutic and pharmacological? The first option was tempting, since lithium differed radically from other psychotropic drugs, and a study of its mode of action seemed a potentially rewarding enterprise. We did in fact carry out a few studies on lithium effects on brain cortex slice respiration, on sodium transfer across the blood–brain barrier, and on cerebral transmitter amine turnover. However, I felt that our unit did not have the expertise for more advanced neurochemical work, nor were we in possession of the equipment necessary for doing such work on a larger scale.

Our research unit was located in a mental hospital, and this offered opportunities for carrying out clinical and experimental work at the same time and on related topics. Clinical observations were followed by animal work, in which conditions could be more stringent and dosages larger. Animal studies yielded pointers for the clinical use of lithium. On more than one occasion this interaction has borne fruit. As a single example may be mentioned the discovery that treatment with diuretics may result in lowering of the lithium clearance, first observed in rats, then confirmed in hypertonic patients treated with diuretics, and finally utilised in the guidelines for psychiatric lithium treatment.[28]

This, then, was to be the pattern of the investigations pursued by the Aarhus group led by Mogens Schou – a primarily clinical approach with supportive animal work. The animal work which followed the 1954 study led to a series of three articles[29] on different aspects of lithium physiology. In rats, toxic effects and renal elimination were studied, and information obtained on the way in which lithium divided itself between serum and tissues. The stimulus for the animal work was, according to Schou,[30] the brief footnote added by G. Masson[31] to the 1949 article of Corcoran, Taylor and Page on salt substitute poisoning.[32] The culmination of this phase of Schou's work was the publication, in 1957, of a detailed review of lithium pharmacology and toxicology, which contained virtually all that was at that time known about the biology of the lithium ion. In the end, however, Schou decided to keep the animal work to a minimum and to concentrate on the clinical studies with which he felt most at home. The decision to concentrate on clinical studies, however, whilst paying handsome dividends, was also to lead Schou and several of his collaborators into a prolonged, and at times bitter, controversy.

Lithium against depression: the discovery of lithium prophylaxis

Upon re-examining the records of patients treated with lithium over a two-year period, Schou noted that one man had responded not only with a reduction in manic episodes but with some attenuation of recurrent depressive episodes too. Perhaps lithium was also effective as an antidepressant? After all, since mania and depression occurred together in the same patient it was not implausible to suppose that even though the two states were symptomatically different there might be some common features in the control mechanisms underlying each. If lithium produced at least part of its therapeutic effect by acting on such mechanisms then it was possible that depression occurring in association with manic episodes might also be lithium-responsive. A double-blind trial was started but soon abandoned; the results were equivocal and failed to lend any clear support to an antidepressive property for lithium salts.

At this point, another figure came into the story: Poul Christian Baastrup, also a psychiatrist, read the report published in 1955[33] by Mogens Schou and his colleagues, and his interest was immediately aroused. When, in 1957, Baastrup had the opportunity to carry out a clinical trial on lithium at the State Hospital in Vordingborg, he decided to take a closer look at the suggestion that lithium had a specific effect on the excitation of manic episodes. Over the next two years he treated fifty-six patients with lithium, confirming Schou's observations that the therapeutic benefits were confined to mania and were not evident on other states of excitation.

Something else, however, emerged from Baastrup's study:

I also found that when lithium was given continuously to manic–depressive patients who had been in hospital for years their condition improved so much that at least some of them could be moved from the closed wards to the open. The result of the trial was presented at a staff meeting in April 1960.[34]

As part of the trial, I conducted a follow-up examination on patients who had been discharged from hospital. After a short course of treatment at the out-patient clinic, they had been asked to stop taking lithium. There were two reasons for this examination: firstly, to make sure that patients did not continue to take lithium without the check-ups, and secondly, to see if lithium treatment had caused any undesirable late side effects or other complications. The result was hair-raising. Eight patients, all with a bipolar course, had continued to take lithium and two of them had even bestowed these 'miracle pills' upon manic–depressive relatives. None of these people had had any kind of check-up, of course. Their reason for continuing the treatment in spite of our agreement was consistent: all of them said that continuous lithium treatment *prevented psychotic relapse*. These patients had had many psychotic episodes over a number of years (mean 12 years, range 3–25 years); from their own experiences they understood clearly their chances of relapse. I can still remember with what mixed and conflicting emotions I faced these eight patients. On the one hand, they had broken a definite agreement and exposed themselves to incalculable and indeterminate risks for which I was responsible. On the other hand, their gratitude at the results was so overwhelming and undeserved. But their claim, however convincing it might seem, could not be right? It did at least deserve to be refuted![35]

It is intriguing to compare the almost chance nature of this observation with that of Cade's original discovery. Like Cade, Baastrup did not let the opportunity slip. Having been unexpectedly presented with a valuable piece of free information, Baastrup did not hesitate to follow it up:

I decided to carry out a retrospective study over a period of three years on high-risk patients who at that time were on lithium. The claim that lithium had a prophylactic effect on psychosis had to be tested. In case the result of the retrospective study was positive, against my expectations, I decided to select a group of high-risk manic–depressive patients for a parallel prospective trial.[36]

The results of the retrospective trial were published in 1964 in *Comprehensive Psychiatry*.[37] The article was quite short – only three pages of text – but had ten pages of clinical case records in diagram form: the results were perfectly clear – lithium did indeed have prophylactic effects against recurrences of depressive episodes.

At exactly the same time that Poul Christian Baastrup was setting up his first clinical study of lithium (about 1957), another psychiatrist was starting a very similar investigation: Dr G. P. Hartigan,[38] a consultant psychiatrist at St Augustine's Hospital of Canterbury, England, administered lithium carbonate to a small group of twenty patients. Nine of these patients showed chronic or intermittent manic episodes, four had alternating manias and depressions of a less than psychotic nature, whilst the remaining seven[39] showed no manic phases, but only recurrent depressive episodes. Of the seven patients with recurrent depression, five responded to prophylactic lithium treatment.

Hartigan did not immediately publish his findings, though he spoke about them to a meeting of the Southeastern Branch of the Royal Medico-psychological Society in 1959,[40] giving a presentation which was at once informative, entertaining, witty, and almost totally inaccurate in its description of the history of lithium therapy up to that time. This hitherto unpublished paper is now printed in full in the Appendix (pp. 183–87).

Hartigan was aware of Mogens Schou's study which had been published five years earlier[41] and so he wrote to Schou in 1960 to give details of his new findings.

> I am venturing to send you a copy of a paper ... that I read to a medical society last year. I do not think it publishable, but there are some observations which I think may be of interest to you, particularly those dealing with the prophylaxis of recurrent depression.[42]

Schou did indeed find it of considerable interest and wrote back to Hartigan[43] congratulating him on his 'vivid and entertaining account' of his experiences with lithium. Schou added that he failed to see why Hartigan's paper should not be published, commenting that it would be 'a pity if these original observations and very convincing case histories were not brought to the attention of a larger group of psychiatrists'.[44]

At about the same time Poul Christian Baastrup also wrote to Schou about *his* results. Schou recognised the important implications of these two independent but identical sets of findings but neither Baastrup nor Hartigan were particularly interested in securing early publication of their findings. Neither had published previously and both evidently felt that their observations were insufficiently systematic to warrant formal presentation.[45]

About a year after receiving Hartigan's first letter, Schou wrote to Hartigan[46] to say that he would be in England in February 1962 for a short visit and would like, if possible, to meet Hartigan to discuss 'common lithium interests and experiences'. Hartigan welcomed the opportunity, and the two met in Canterbury towards the end of February 1962. Schou was able to see Hartigan's patients at first hand. According to Schou, these, though few in number, were very striking, including individuals who had experienced recurrent depressions over a considerable number of years but who had been free of such episodes throughout their two years on lithium therapy.[47] On his return to Denmark, Schou wrote again[48] to Hartigan to thank him for his hospitality, and to state again his conviction that Hartigan's observations were of the greatest importance.

> I must say that I found the five cases presented very convincing. I have told my clinical colleagues about these patients, and we shall be on the look-out for patients who might fall in the category that seems to profit from preventive lithium treatment. May I once more urge you to publish your experiences; I consider them much too valuable to be hidden in a drawer.[49]

Hartigan, however, failed to be moved by this plea. Schou recalls[50] that Hartigan had appeared to him to be rather shy and self-effacing, and this was certainly reflected in his reluctance to make his observations public. Seven months later, Schou wrote again:[51]

> I know that you were not very eager about this [the publication of the prophylaxis observations] and felt your material was too small to convince anybody. I do not agree with you there. . . .
> If you have not yet done it, please consider again publishing a report. There comes a point where people may become suspicious if I continue referring to the 'unpublished observations' and 'personal communication' from G. P. Hartigan while this person himself remains silent![52]

Schou added the suggestion that Hartigan should send an account of the findings to Dr Eliot Slater, editor of the *Journal of Mental Science*; Schou felt that Slater would probably be kindly disposed towards a submission from Hartigan, being already convinced of the advantages of lithium in the treatment of chronic mania.

This time Hartigan was persuaded and he sent a copy of the original lecture to Slater, 'and if he thinks anything of it, I must bestir myself to get into print'.[53] Over a month passed, and Hartigan received no response to his submission. 'I have heard nothing further from Slater', he wrote to Schou,[54] but indicated now his firm resolve to organise the material into a publishable form: 'I shall therefore commit myself to publication fairly soon if I can get any misguided editor to accept it'.[55]

Eventually, Hartigan heard from Slater that a completely rewritten version of Hartigan's paper might be acceptable for publication in the *British Journal of Psychiatry*, and towards the end of 1962 the draft of the new article was completed and sent to Schou for his comments.[56] Early in 1963 it appeared in print.[57]

In the spring of that year Baastrup received from Schou a copy of Hartigan's paper[58] and when he published his own findings the following year[59] he made reference to Hartigan's work.

Whilst Hartigan must therefore clearly be accorded priority in reporting the results of clinical trials demonstrating the prophylactic efficacy of lithium against recurrent endogenous depression, there can equally be no doubt that Hartigan and Baastrup reached this conclusion quite independently and simultaneously.

The role of Mogens Schou in the years when lithium was being formulated as a prophylactic antidepressant was threefold. In the first place, as an encourager and stimulator he was able to persuade both Hartigan and Baastrup of the need to make their findings available to a wide public.[60] As a clinician already convinced of the therapeutic efficacy of lithium against mania, Schou was well placed to appreciate the importance of the finding that depressive states might also, under some circumstances, respond to lithium treatment, and he was therefore quick to identify the subject as one to be actively pursued. As a theoretician, Schou was able to put together the evidence about the clinical actions of lithium in a way which invited comment on, and stimulated interest in, the clinical effectiveness of lithium – this he did in an article published in 1963,[61] in which he introduced the term 'normothymotics'[62] to describe a group of drugs (exemplified by lithium and imipramine) which 'normalised' a psychiatric state by exerting a specific action against the pathological lesion underlying the disease state. The background to this article is quite interesting. Early in September 1962, Schou heard a talk given at a psychiatric meeting in Munich[63] by Professor Haruo Akimoto of Tokyo in which it was reported that manic patients had been treated with the antidepressant drug imipramine with very good results. Schou related this to his knowledge – based on the work of Hartigan and Baastrup – that lithium acted against both phases of manic–depressive psychosis, and hypothesised that, despite the fact that the two substances were clearly chemically quite different, lithium and imipramine might share a common mode of action therapeutically. He drew some support for this view from the additional fact that imipramine and its derivatives produced certain characteristic electrocardiographic effects in a number of patients, effects which seemed to be reproduced by lithium but not by other drugs.[64]

Schou developed his arguments in a manuscript which was submitted to the *Lancet* on the advice of Eliot Slater, but which the *Lancet* rejected. Slater subsequently accepted it for the *British Journal of Psychiatry*.[65]

Personal motives

The decision which any investigator makes to follow one line of study rather than another is necessarily a complex one and difficult to analyse, even for the investigator himself. Frequently, factors may enter into the decision which have little to do with either logic or science but which are, to the investigator, of equal importance. In the case of Mogens Schou, interest in the general topic of affective disorders was in large measure prompted by the occurrence of a number of instances of manic–depression within his own family. In a letter which he sent to Hartigan in 1961,[66] to ask whether any further clinical data had been obtained, Schou broached the matter of the familial link.

I am asking about this not only out of interest in the use of lithium in psychiatry; but also because one of my brothers has been suffering from depressions that recur with great regularity.[67]

Hartigan replied[68] that he thought that 'in your brother's case it should be well worth trying'. Schou did so, with dramatic success: following the institution of lithium therapy, his brother had no further depressive relapses.

When, in 1981, Schou received an honorary doctorate from the University of Aix-Marseille, he gave an address in which he outlined the extent to which his brother's improvement had hardened his resolve to discover as much as possible about lithium therapy.

From the age of twenty he suffered from repeated attacks of depression, which periodically made him unable, in spite of high intelligence, to carry out his chosen profession. The attacks usually lasted some months, and then disappeared, but they reappeared again and again, year after year, inevitably. Then, about 14 years ago, he was started on maintenance treatment with lithium, and since then he has not had a single depressive relapse. He still needs to take the medicine to keep the disease under control, but functionally he is a cured man. You will understand what such a change meant to himself and to his wife and children, and how much of a miracle it appeared to us in the family. Fear of the future has been replaced by confidence and new hope.[69]

Early investigations of prophylaxis

As a result of his exchange of letters with both Hartigan and Baastrup, Schou began to keep in close contact with Baastrup, realising that such a pooling of resources and ideas could lead to a more accurate evaluation of the clinical potential of lithium. The first result of their cooperation was the joint publication, in 1967, of the results obtained from Baastrup's prospective study of high-risk manic–depressive patients who had been put on lithium six and a half years earlier. Baastrup had made a preliminary report of the findings in 1966 at a meeting of the Danish Psychiatric Association; the full report appeared the following year in the *Archives of General Psychiatry*.[70] According to this report, relapses (affective episodes) occurred in patients significantly less frequently during lithium treatment than before such treatment, and moreover the total duration of psychosis was also markedly reduced. The nature of the cooperation between Baastrup and Schou was clearly indicated: collection of the clinical data was ascribed to Baastrup, whilst 'the definition of the material and its evaluation and presentation are the result of a collaboration between the authors'.[71]

Baastrup and Schou were well aware that their findings were only preliminary and that the experimental design which had been used was potentially subject to certain criticisms. In particular, the conclusions which had been drawn from the study were based on a comparison of patients' before-treatment relapse rates with their after-treatment relapse rates, and this necessarily involved the assumption that if treatment had *not* been given the relapse rate would have been maintained at (at least) the same level. Such an assumption might or might not be justified. Fortunately, there was work already in progress which was directed at just this question. Professor Jules Angst of Zurich University Psychiatric Clinic had been carrying out investigations since about 1964 on the time-course of affective disorders, in association with Dr Paul Weis (a statistician), and had developed a multiple regression model for the analysis of the course of affective and schizo-affective disorders. At a meeting in Haiti in April 1966,[72] Schou informed Angst of the prophylactic properties of lithium and Angst subsequently started – in Zurich – to use lithium as a prophylactic agent. Angst joined his efforts with those of Paul Grof (of Prague), and by 1969 the group had collected data on 979 cases of affective disorder and a total of 2216 mood cycles. The most important result of this work, as far as Baastrup and Schou were concerned, was clear confirmation that the logical basis of their clinical trial had been sound. As Angst and his colleagues[73] put it:

> On average endogenous affective psychoses show a regular decrease in the length of the cycles with increasing number of episodes. If one cuts the course of an affective psychosis at any time, one has to compare identical spaces of time on both sides of this cut. One can expect that there will be more episodes after the cut than before.[74]

They found evidence for a prophylactic effect of lithium but not of imipramine. The final application of the multiple regression model was the basis of the joint report of the Danish, Swiss and Czech investigators. The pooled data were analysed in Switzerland and a joint report was submitted, under a single pseudonym, to the International Anna-Monika-Stiftung: it took the first prize. This long report was subsequently split into several shorter articles which were published in the *British Journal of Psychiatry*.[75]

It would be quite wrong to give the impression that whilst Hartigan, Baastrup and Schou were pursuing their investigations of lithium prophylaxis nothing else was going on in the field of lithium research. On the contrary, according to an analysis by Kline[76] of the early clinical reports published on lithium, there were details given between 1959 and 1968 (inclusive) of in excess of 1400 patients treated with lithium, even excluding those reported by Baastrup and Schou. In general, these reports, which came from many different investigators based in a wide variety of countries, were favourable in their assessment of lithium as an antimanic agent, and some reports confirmed Baastrup and Schou's finding of a prophylactic action against recurrent depression. This culminated in the publication by Schou of a long and detailed review of lithium usage[77] in which the evidence was presented in a clear and persuasive manner. This review, which was to become, over the next ten years, the most extensively quoted article on the subject of lithium therapy, was powerfully influential in extending the use of lithium throughout the world.

By 1968 there was, therefore, a sizeable body of opinion which regarded lithium as a useful drug in psychiatric practice. There was also, however, growing opposition. Poul Christian Baastrup, for example, has referred to 'considerable opposition to the use of continuous lithium treatment, not least from academics, although this opposition was not supported by criticism of our work ....'[78] Asked to give more details of the resistance which he met, Baastrup replied that 'the main point was that both physicians to whom I had a near connection in my daily work and physicians working at the psychiatric clinic in the university of Copenhagen refused to use lithium; straightforward questions were answered in different ways – the treatment was too dangerous, the results published were incredible/untrustworthy/unreliable: the criticisms were never made publicly'.[79]

In Australia, too, Trautner was meeting similar problems. When, in August 1954, Schou sent Trautner a pre-publication copy of the paper which was to appear in *Neurology, Neurosurgery and Psychiatry*,[80] Trautner replied[81] that he and his colleagues were 'very glad to see that you were able to confirm our results, particularly in view of a lot of opposition we meet'. In Trautner's case, it is possible that this opposition was, to some extent, justified because in the early days of lithium therapy, before the guidelines to safe dosage were properly established, there were probably more serious intoxications than were formally recognised. Lithium was felt by many to be a capriciously toxic substance.

Baastrup and Schou, however, were concerned right from the outset to try to avoid toxicity by means of the careful monitoring of serum lithium levels. They showed, indeed, considerable concern about the whole question of lithium intoxication and much of their early work was directed towards understanding it and towards devising techniques for either minimising the chances of its occurrence or treating it rapidly and effectively when it did occur. Despite this, the opponents of lithium therapy began to make their views apparent. For the most part this manifested itself as minor, but irritating, obstructions within the hospital system: such things, whilst annoying, were not particularly serious and the lithium pioneers could afford to take the difficulties in their stride in the hope that, with time, even those who doubted the efficacy of lithium could not help but eventually be converted by the weight of steadily accumulating clinical evidence. Whilst this did eventually come about, the change was slower than anyone in the early 1960s could have predicted: towards the end of that decade a challenge was mounted in the pages of the *Lancet* to the whole basis of lithium therapy, and the intense controversy to which this gave rise was to last for over three years.[82]

Plates I to XVIII

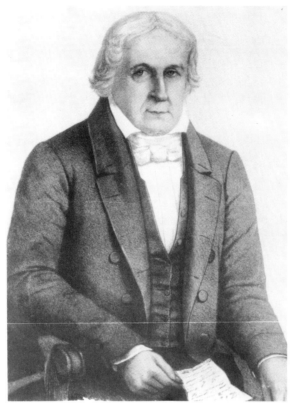

Plate I   Joze Bonifacio de Andrada e Silva (1763–1838), discoverer of spodumene and petalite, two ores of lithium. Reproduced by courtesy of the Government of Brazil.

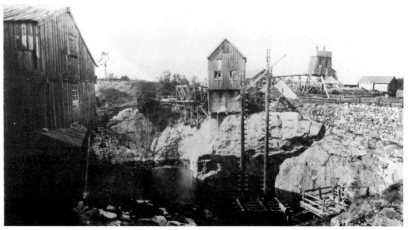

Plate II   Iron ore mine on the island of Utö, site of the discovery of spodumene and petalite in 1800. Reproduced by courtesy of the Tekniska Museet, Stockholm, Sweden.

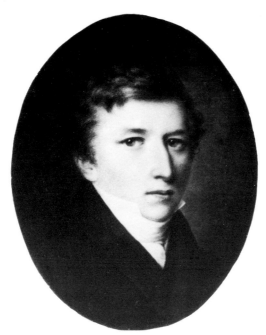

Plate III   Johan August Arfwedson (1792–1841) who identified the presence of a new element in petalite. Reproduced by courtesy of the Stockholm University Library from the portrait collection in the Royal Swedish Academy of Sciences.

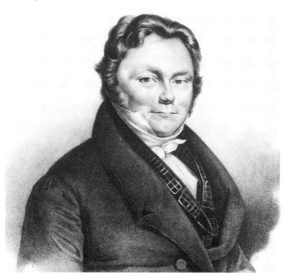

Plate IV   Baron Jons Jacob Berzelius (1779–1848) in whose laboratory lithium was first identified and who gave the new element its name. Reproduced by courtesy of the Stockholm University Library from the portrait collection in the Royal Swedish Academy of Sciences.

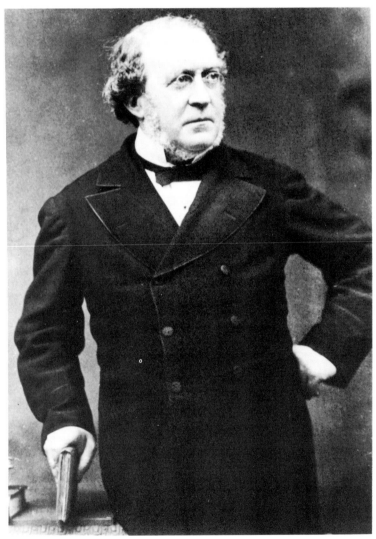

Plate V   Sir Alfred Baring Garrod, FRS (1819–1907) who proposed the use of lithium salts in the treatment of gout. Reproduced by courtesy of the Royal College of Physicians, London.

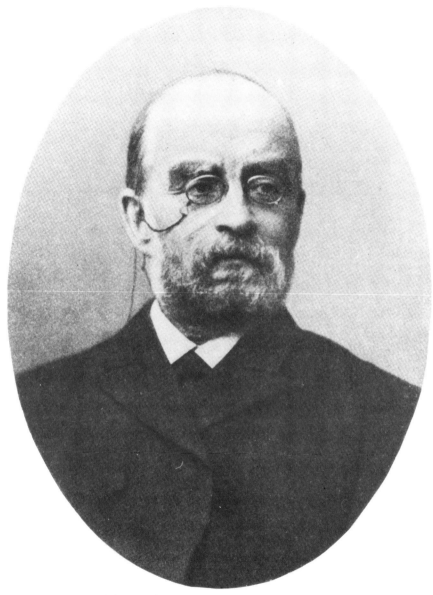

Plate VI   Carl Lange (1834–1900) who was probably the first to use
lithium salts systematically in the prophylactic treatment of depression.

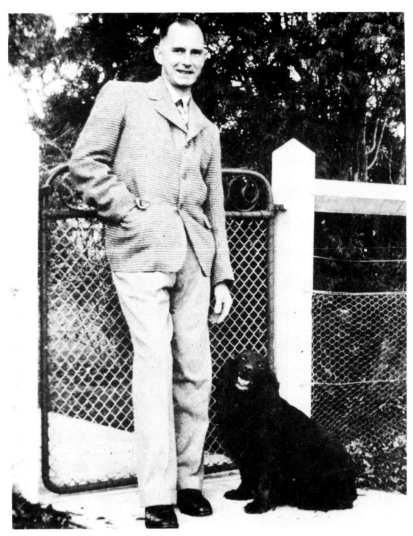

Plate VII John Frederick Joseph Cade (1912–1980), the modern discoverer of the antimanic action of lithium. This photograph was taken when Cade was Medical Superintendent at Bundoora. Reproduced by courtesy of Dr John Cade Jr, from a print kindly supplied by Dr H. D. Attwood of the Medical History Unit, University of Melbourne.

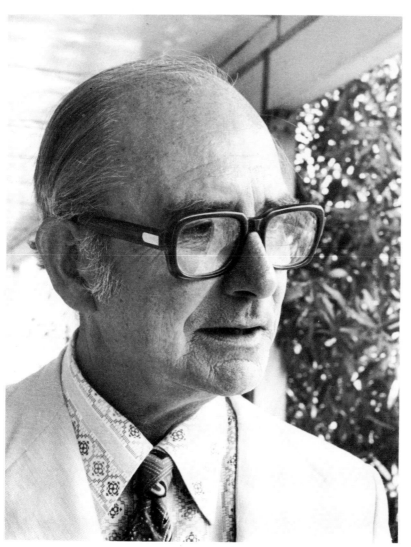

Plate VIII   John Cade in later life.

W.B.   aet. 51.

Chronic mania of about 5 yrs duration. Fair but temporary improvement after E.C.T. 2 yrs ago. Since Nov. '46 has completely reverted to his usual state – noisy, restless, untidy & mischievous.

29/3/48. Commenced lithium citrate mixture gr x tds. After a few days increased to gr xx tds & then for a few days to gr xl tds – commenced to vomit & c/o nocturnal enuresis. Mental state improving. Dosage reduced & still sensitive, so discontinued & replaced with capsules of Li_2CO_3 gr v. b.d.

5/5/48. Has been in A ward for about 10 days, and after steadily settling down, now has appeared perfectly normal both to my observation & that of his relatives for over a week. Continues on Li_2CO_3 gr v b.d. in capsules.

14/5/48. Continues well   20/5/48. Continues well.

29/5/48. A little unsettled today. Discontented that he has not been able to go home (housing difficulty). Li_2CO_3 incr. to gr x tds.

30/5/48. Settled down again.
31/6/48. Li_2CO_3 reduced to gr v. tds. Well.   7/6/48. Well.

9/6/48. Li_2CO_3 incr. to gr x tds.

14/6/48. Very well. More self confidence   20/6/48. S.Q.

25/6/48. O.T.L. for week end. Improved still further.

29/6/48. Very well. Li_2CO_3 reduced to gr v tds.

2/7/48. O.T.L. 5 days   8/7/48. R.T.L. – v. well.

9/7/48. On indefinite T.L. To report in fortnight. Continuing c̄ Li_2CO_3 gr v tds.

24/7/48. Seen this A.M. V. well. Has been at work since last wk., back c̄ old firm. Li_2CO_3 reduced to gr v b.d. To report in 4 wks.

11/9/48. Seen today. Very well mentally & continues at work. Off colour for a few days c̄ dyspepsia.

13/11/48. Seen today. Well. Working. Discontinued Li_2CO_3 about 6/52 ago. Some vomiting recently – put on mist. by local M.O. & no trouble since. Has lost no wt. & sleeping extremely well. To report in 3/12.

24/11/48. S. in law in letter states has become excitable & argumentative after trivial row last Sun. 21/11. Pt. written to, to come out for interview on 27/11 & recommence Li_2CO_3.

29/11/48. Seen this A.M. – quiet & rational but a bit uneasy. To recommence Li_2CO_3 gr x tds 7 days, gr v tds 7 days, then gr v. b.d.

15/12/48. S. in law writes – irritable, not taking med. regularly.

Plate IX   Two of John Cade's case record cards giving details of his first patient (W.B.) to receive lithium treatment. Reproduced by courtesy of the University of Melbourne.

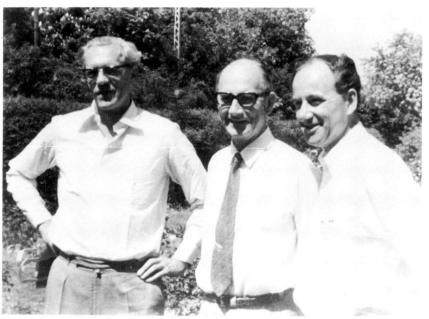

Plate X   Poul Christian Baastrup, John Cade and Mogens Schou, the three fathers of modern lithium therapy.

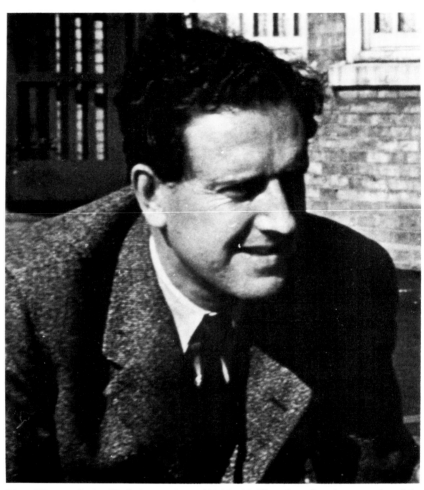

Plate XI   G. P. (Toby) Hartigan (1917–1968), who, simultaneously with, but independently of, Poul Christian Baastrup, identified the prophylactic properties of lithium against recurrent depression.

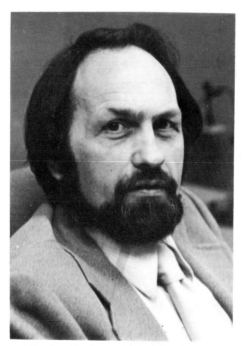

Plate XII   Barry Blackwell who, with Michael Shepherd, labelled lithium prophylaxis 'a therapeutic myth'.

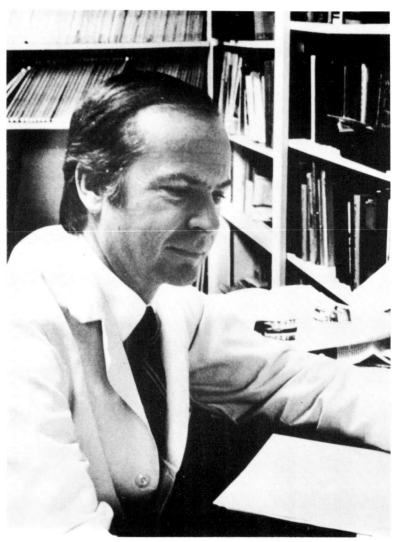

Plate XIII   Ronald R. Fieve who conducted the earliest clinical trials of lithium in the USA.

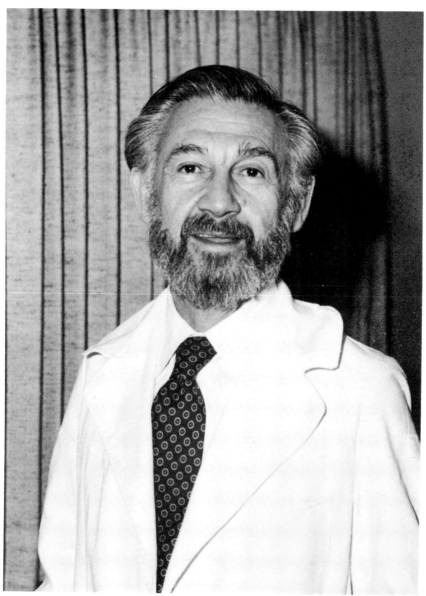

Plate XIV   Samuel Gershon who played a major role in extending
Australian experience of lithium therapy to the USA.

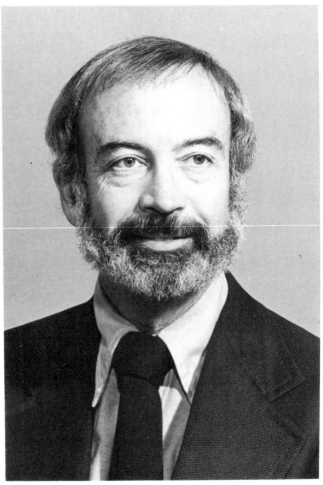

Plate XV   Joe Tupin who first obtained official approval in the USA to investigate lithium therapy.

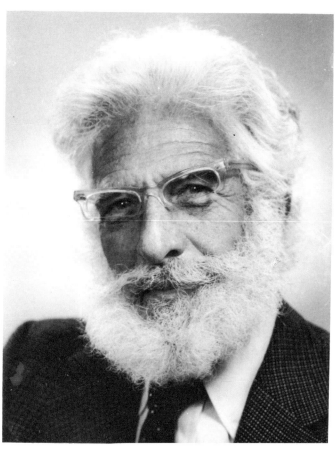

Plate XVI   Nathan S. Kline was a major force in developing lithium therapy in the USA. He died in February 1983.

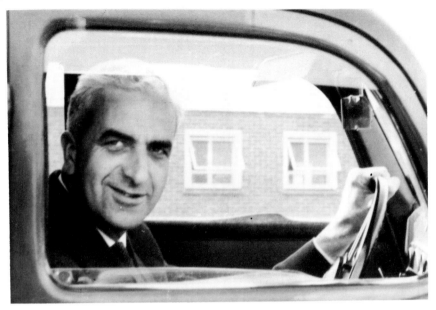

Plate XVII   David Rice, author of the first British publication on the antimanic action of lithium.

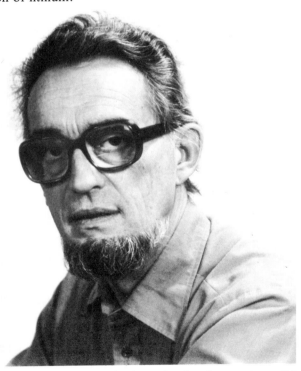

Plate XVIII   Amdi Amdisen, who has stimulated awareness of the value of serum lithium estimation.

7

The therapeutic myth

The attack on lithium prophylaxis

In 1967, a young doctor by the name of Barry Blackwell completed his training in both psychiatry and pharmacology at the Maudsley Hospital in London. He was offered, and accepted, a place as a Research Fellow at the Maudsley, and worked for the next year with Professor Michael Shepherd who was then Professor of Epidemiological Psychiatry.[1] At that time, the claims for lithium prophylaxis were beginning to be loudly heard, and Blackwell's interest in the topic was immediately aroused. He and Shepherd examined the data that were available and came to the conclusion that the claims for prophylactic efficacy were simply not supported by the evidence. They presented their argument in an article entitled 'Prophylactic lithium: another therapeutic myth?' which was published in the *Lancet* on 4 May 1968.[2]

The article was a hard-hitting one. The primary focus of the attack was the 1967 article by Poul Christian Baastrup and Mogens Schou[3] in which Baastrup's clinical data had been presented, 'since the evidence for a "prophylactic" action of lithium depends on this key paper'.[4] The criticisms levelled against Baastrup and Schou's findings fell under four headings. In the first place, Blackwell and Shepherd argued that the criteria used for including patients in the study could have led to the inappropriate inclusion of up to a quarter of the total cases considered: such patients, they argued, might actually have been suffering from non-recurrent affective disorders, the apparent periodicity being due rather to 'fragmentation' of the illness by the use of electroconvulsive therapy or antidepressant drugs. By the time that lithium was introduced, these patients were effectively cured anyway.

Secondly, the criteria for establishing successful prophylaxis were felt not to have been applied with sufficient rigour. Since this represents the core of the case against Baastrup and Schou, the argument is presented in full:

Demonstration of prophylaxis demands that the patient remains well both during treatment and for a longer period than can be attributed to spontaneous remission. Several patients failed to meet these requirements. 20 patients relapsed, 5 of whom seem to have become worse during treatment. . . . The apparent benefit derived from lithium can be linked to the relatively short follow-up period. In 17 patients the remission during lithium therapy was shorter than had previously occurred without lithium. . . . In addition, 15 patients who had been ill before the treatment period had remissions lasting well into it and exceeding the length of the lithium-induced remission. The null hypothesis that patients remain equally well with or without lithium would mean that half the 88 patients could be expected to have illness-free intervals equal to lithium-induced remissions. Since the difference between this hypothetical 44 and the observed 32 is not significant ($\chi^2 = 2.8021$; $p = 0.1$), the value of lithium in maintaining wellbeing remains unproven.

Altogether, a prophylactic action of lithium is doubtful in no fewer than 55 cases. Of the original 88 patients 22 were doubtfully recurrent; 5 remained ill on treatment, and 15 relapsed on it; 32 patients underwent spontaneous remissions longer than those attributable to lithium, 17 of these being apparent and 15 inferred from the data. Only 33 (21 per cent) remained with a clearly satisfactory outcome suggestive of a 'prophylactic' action due to lithium.[5]

The third objection related to the evaluation of the clinical results. Blackwell and Shepherd argued that 'the statistical method chosen by Baastrup and Schou weights the facts in favour of their hypothesis'.[6] Using a series of examples, Blackwell and Shepherd tried to show that the choice of indices such as the number of relapses before and after lithium, and the number of months' illness per year, biased the findings in favour of finding a prophylactic effect. In addition, the selection of patients who had successfully completed one year's continuous lithium therapy would, it was claimed, effectively exclude some seriously relapsing patients as well as patients who discontinued therapy.

Finally, Blackwell and Shepherd were not prepared to accept the justification for an open, as distinct from a double-blind, trial, despite the assertions by Baastrup and Schou that no observer bias had entered into their study.

They used an 'open' method to evaluate a therapy for which they have been enthusiastic advocates for several years. In such circumstances patients are inevitably given a quality of care and follow-up superior to any they have experienced before, especially when they receive a potent drug such as lithium which necessitates exhortations to take regular medication and attend frequently for electrolyte estimations. A clinician committed to the ideal of 'prophylaxis' will be prepared to manipulate dosage and give adjunctive out-patient support to forestall admission, itself the main criterion of success or failure.[7]

This was certainly very blunt and to the point, and the article made a considerable impact. As Blackwell later said, 'our article was (as you might imagine) not very kindly received by researchers in the field and was felt to be a personal attack on Schou's scholarly integrity'. It is not, however, easy to understand Blackwell's further comment about the article: 'My impression is that it was dealt with by studied avoidance – a kind of academic cold shoulder',[8] since Baastrup and Schou published a trenchant and detailed riposte in the *Lancet* only one month after the appearance of Blackwell and Shepherd's attack.[9] In their refutation of the criticisms made of their work, they dealt with the four points on which Blackwell and Shepherd had placed greatest emphasis.

The suggestion that pre-lithium treatment with ECT or other drugs might have 'fragmented' single illnesses so as to mimic recurrent conditions was countered by noting that relapses occurring during lithium treatment were also treated by these other procedures, and that any possible fragmentation effect would be equally distributed before and during lithium therapy. The exclusion of patients who did not complete the year's treatment with lithium was noted as not biasing the data in favour of lithium prophylaxis, but actually acting *against* it, since such patients tended to be the ones who had actually benefited most from the treatment:

> They had been without relapse for a period of months and felt they could do without further medication.... Any bias introduced by these exclusions would tend to weight the evidence *against* the notion of lithium prophylaxis.[10]

The argument that the statistical analysis was at fault was dismissed as 'difficult to comprehend' on the grounds that the original analysis was based on all the eighty-eight patients in the investigation, whilst Blackwell and Shepherd had selected just three.

As far as the criteria for prophylaxis were concerned, Baastrup and Schou pointed to a fundamental flaw in the argument put forward by Blackwell and Shepherd who had taken the end of the follow-up period as being the start of a relapse. 'It comes as no surprise', Baastrup and Schou added, 'that they fail to obtain statistical significance with data so grossly misinterpreted'.[11]

Effects of observer bias, as suggested by Blackwell and Shepherd, were refuted:

> A study of our original paper will reveal that mood changes were counted as relapses only when they were sufficiently severe to necessitate regular supervision in the home or admission to a mental hospital. The decisions concerning these measures were not made by us; recording of relapses was therefore uninfluenced by possible investigator bias. Blackwell and Shepherd further insinuate that we manipulated dosages to forestall admission. It must be noted that any departure from the fixed-dosage

schedule took place under clearly specified circumstances; dosages were increased only after patients had suffered relapse, not to forestall it'.[12]

By these and other arguments, Baastrup and Schou dealt with all the objections which Blackwell and Shepherd had raised, but controversies of whatever nature are rarely so easily resolved and opinion about the therapeutic applications of lithium became sharply divided amongst psychiatrists. There were those who came out strongly in favour of Baastrup and Schou, quoting their own clinical experience and clinical trial results. From Yorkshire in England, for example, Dr Roy Hullin and his colleagues wrote to the *Lancet* to give a preliminary report of successful lithium prophylaxis in forty patients.[13] The Danish findings were so well received amongst Scandinavian psychiatrists that it actually became rather difficult to carry out proper clinical trials, as Björn Laurell and Jan-Otto Ottosson found.[14] After setting up a double-blind study of lithium, they felt them-selves forced to abandon it at an early stage because of 'the publicity that lithium has been given in Sweden, where most psychiatrists believe that its value far outweighs its risks in severe recurrent affective psychoses'.[15] An additional problem was that their patients had come to hear about the value of lithium and specifically requested that it should be given. Laurell and Ottosson felt keenly the ethical problem of not giving these patients lithium in order to put them in a control group. As they said:

> In our opinion, it is now too late to make a study in Sweden in which a simultaneous control group is not given lithium. The problem might be less in countries where knowledge of lithium is more limited or the psychological conditions different.[16]

On the other hand, Drs Ronald Fieve and Stanley Platman in the USA noted[17] that their own double-blind study had shown that lithium 'does not appear to alter the frequency of depressive attacks, and showed at best a mild tendency to decrease depressive scores . . . over time'.[18] Fieve and Platman concluded that 'it might be injurious to claim at this point that lithium is effective as an antidepressant, or as a prophylactic for recurrent depression per se'.[19]

A further objection to the Danish study came from Dr Malcolm Lader of University College, London. In a letter to the *Lancet*[20] shortly after Baastrup and Schou's rebuttal of Blackwell and Shepherd's criticisms, Lader reopened the question of the appropriateness of the statistical analyses performed in support of the conclusion that lithium prophylaxis had occurred. One point in particular was raised: the null hypothesis that, if treatment by lithium were without effect, there would be equal probabilities of increase and decrease of relapse rate under lithium, was said to be approp-riate only if each patient could have expected to get the same number of attacks in the year following institution of lithium as had occurred in the year before. 'This', said Lader, 'is manifestly absurd assuming as it does that once a patient has had two or more psychotic attacks he will continue to have them indefinitely',[21] and he added that 'most psychiatrists would agree that it is impossible to predict with any degree of certainty the course of an illness of this type'.[22] That, however, was exactly what *had* been predicted by Jules Angst and his colleagues[23] and Baastrup and Schou were not slow to point this out.[24]

Blackwell versus Kline: the Cinderella letters

Despite the spirited defence mounted by Baastrup and Schou, and others (such as Dr William Sargant[25] who felt that statistical arguments had been allowed to get out of hand and to obtrude upon clinical commonsense), Barry Blackwell was not prepared to let the matter drop. His opportunity came when Dr Nathan Kline wrote an editorial entitled 'Lithium comes into its own' in the October 1968 issue of the *American Journal of Psychiatry*,[26] in which he stated that 'lithium, the 20-year old Cinderella of psychophar-macology, is at last receiving her sovereign due'.[27] Kline referred to the exchange which had occurred in the pages of the *Lancet* that year, and recalled that after Baastrup and Schou had made their reply a meeting had been arranged at a symposium of the Royal Medicopsychological Association at which 'all of the principals plus a few other interested persons were scheduled to appear'.[28] The meeting, which was held in Plymouth in July 1968, appears to have been something of a disaster; according to Kline, Michael Shepherd was unable to attend because of a prior engagement and a misunderstanding over the date, and Schou was ill. Barry Blackwell was there, however, and as Kline put it 'led off his own presentation with the clear statement that he had never treated a single patient with lithium'.[29] This was too much for Blackwell who sent a letter to the editor of the *American Journal of Psychiatry* in which his attack on Kline was only thinly masked with irony:

Sir, The editorial 'Lithium comes into its own' by Dr Nathan S. Kline ... will be highly prized by collectors of original enthusiasm tempered by subsequent experience. Only time will show whether your author's eulogy earns him the fate his analogy deserves – to join Cinderella's fairy godmother in the pages of mythology. To transform 'just plain old lithium' into the elixir of life on the evidence available is an achievement second only to converting a pumpkin into a stagecoach.

Doubtless, Dr Kline's recollections of the Royal Medicopsychological Association meeting in Plymouth are as inexact as mine are, although both merit consideration. I recall his exuberant certainty that clinical impression could replace controlled evaluation, a fact your readers may take into account when weighing the evidence. ...

Before joining the lithium crowd, your readers might ponder the lessons to be learned from the honest, well-intentioned enthusiasts who championed the ducking stool, purging, bleeding, and even insulin. They and their patients learned the long, hard way, the need for proper controlled evaluation of therapy in psychiatry.

I have still not treated a patient with lithium, but I hope I can evaluate evidence. This common dilemma confronts all of us who work in research, industry, or even the Food and Drug Administration. A little detachment may perhaps be of assistance.[30]

Kline's reply also combined humour with acidity:

Sir, Dr Blackwell's delightful letter reads as though it were written by one of Cinderella's spiteful sisters. Lithium is more like the lost slipper than the pumpkin-stagecoach. It isn't meant for everyone, but when it does fit, there actually is a fairy story quality about it.

In view of the lack of 'proper controlled evaluation of therapy' in all areas of medicine prior to twenty or thirty years ago, it is really most disconcerting to note the discovery of quinine, digitalis, opiates, aspirin, and a few hundred other useful pharmaceuticals. There is even a feeling of faint personal familiarity with Dr Blackwell's 'warning' which reminds me of some of the caveats concerning the introduction of both the antipsychotic and antidepressant agents. Of course it may also be that Dr Blackwell is also not convinced that any of these drugs have been demonstrated to be of use.

The real problem would seem to be the relatively medieval mathematical model upon which Dr Blackwell is 'hung-up'. Its application in most cases constitutes a triumph of technique over purpose. Fortunately it now appears that most of us (like the hero of *Le Bourgeois Gentilhomme*: 'Good Heavens! For more than forty years I have been speaking prose without knowing it.' Act II, scene 4) have been using the Baysian approach without being aware of how astute we were. As the mathematical model becomes more clearly defined, it is evident that the clinician was correct when he insisted that his approach was more meaningful and appropriate than models based upon Fisherian statistics. Montesquieu was thus correct when he stated 'A good doctor should know a little about everything – even medicine'.[31]

A further attack by Blackwell

Blackwell remained undaunted. In November, 1969, he repeated the substance of his earlier attack, with some additional arguments, in *Medical Counterpoint*.[32] In this article, Blackwell struck out in all directions. Once again he referred to Kline's characterisation of lithium 'as a Cinderella waiting patiently by the fireside of psychopharmacology for a Prince Charming he intends to emulate'.[32] Baastrup and Schou were taken to task on the grounds that 'their enthusiasm for lithium is attested by the numbers given it, including pregnant women, and by the attempts made to rationalise treatment failures'.[34] The work of Jules Angst and his group concerning the course of manic depressive illness, on which Baastrup and Schou had defended their decision to compare pre- and post-lithium relapse rates, was also not spared: Blackwell referred to 'considerable shortcomings'[35] in the data.

Blackwell attempted to provide some explanation of why the claims for a prophylactic efficacy of lithium against depression should continue to be pressed in the absence of what, in his opinion, was satisfactory supporting evidence. He considered several possibilities.

In the first place, if lithium were effective only acutely against mania, it would not, in Blackwell's view, have remained of any great psychopharmacological interest, thereby rendering worthless the work of a number of individuals who had invested considerable personal prestige in the subject:

When lithium slipped out of sight again in 1954, several enthusiasts were already espoused to its virtues and continued to search for a use. If this had been confined to the treatment of mania, the compound would have remained in obscurity. Mania is a rare condition, difficult to treat with oral medication and one for which chlorpromazine had already become a safe and reasonably effective remedy. The claim which projected lithium into prominence was that while it was only moderately effective in treating mania and ineffective in depression, it was still capable of suppressing 'mood swings' and preventing affective illnesses from occurring.[36]

Blackwell made no secret of the fact that he was referring to Mogens Schou and Nathan Kline in particular:

In Scandinavia, Schou's whole professional life since 1954 has been dominated by lithium, and he has published over sixty papers on the topic. His persistent refusal to attempt double-blind methodology is partly determined by his strong personal convictions about the drug.

In America, Kline has adopted lithium, repeating the role he previously fulfilled for reserpine and the monoamine oxidase inhibitors of 'convincing the world'.... Kline, like Schou, has not conducted double-blind studies, but retains an exuberant and infectious enthusiasm for prophylactic lithium.[37]

Unlike the original article in the *Lancet* labelling lithium as a 'therapeutic myth', Blackwell's much more detailed *Medical Counterpoint* article failed to arouse any response from Baastrup or Schou. Even when Shepherd repeated[38] the arguments, adding that 'on ethical as well as scientific grounds it would seem improper to publicise such far-reaching claims until the evidence has been established beyond reasonable doubt',[39] no reaction was elicited.

The steady pressure of questioning of the claims made for lithium were, however, having their effect. There grew up a new atmosphere of scepticism about the therapeutic effectiveness of lithium salts. Drs Willie Kai Shull and Joseph Sapira[40] actually went so far as to suggest that the evidence for even an antimanic effect – something which not even Blackwell and Shepherd had seriously challenged – might not be adequate.

The double-blind discontinuation study

By the beginning of 1969 it was clear that, to restore confidence in the idea of lithium prophylaxis, Baastrup and Schou were going to have to go beyond a simple refutation of Blackwell and Shepherd's criticisms, and would need to produce new evidence avoiding the methodological issues which had been the subject of contention. There were, however, a number of problems.

In the first place, Baastrup and Schou felt that the attack which had been made on their work was directed at a personal, as well as scientific, level: this belief made it difficult to see what type of positive response might be most appropriate. It did not help that neither Baastrup nor Schou could understand why a personal element should have entered into the controversy in the first place, if indeed it had.

Schou recalls[41] having met Shepherd in Göttingen, West Germany, shortly after the first results of Baastrup's prospective study had been gathered: he reported eagerly about the prophylactic results, including the successful outcome of his brother's treatment, and he asked Shepherd's opinion about the methodology used. Shepherd did not react positively or negatively, but when he and Schou met at a conference in Spain one month before the appearance of Blackwell and Shepherd's *Lancet* article, Shepherd informed Schou that in collaboration with a colleague he had written a critique of the lithium prophylaxis data. This was all the information given. Nor did either Baastrup or Schou receive a preprint of the critique from Shepherd, or any indication from the editor of the *Lancet* that the article was in press. While one must not lay too much stress on this latter point, it is, nevertheless, worth making since it is a not uncommon editorial practice to refer critical articles to the person or persons being attacked so that they have the opportunity to submit a reply if they so wish.

This, then, was the first barrier to an effective rejoinder by Baastrup and Schou – what was the best strategy to follow, given that the motivation behind what they perceived as a personal element in the attack was by no means clear? As Schou puts it, 'After swallowing a few times, we decided that we had to ignore those aspects of the article which we regarded as not constructive, and to analyse the critique for its good points – those criticisms of methodology which might have some validity.'[42]

That their early study had not been perfect, Schou and Baastrup conceded; that observer bias could have been involved they also accepted as possible in principle but as highly unlikely in practice. It seemed clear that only a rigorously executed double-blind study would suffice to settle the matter. Here, however, the second problem arose, and this time it was a much more serious one.

Schou and Baastrup were '99 per cent convinced'[43] that lithium was prophylactically effective against recurrent depression, and that to deprive their patients of this treatment would be both dangerous and ethically difficult to defend. This difficulty was made all the more poignant by directly affecting Schou personally: his brother who had suffered depression every year since the age of twenty had not had a single recurrence since receiving lithium. 'How *could* I put him, or others like him, in a clinical trial where he would face the possibility of lithium being withdrawn?' Schou asked.[44]

There was, however, another side to the coin, as Baastrup and Schou well realised. Whilst lithium treatment had been taken up throughout continental Europe, and had been generally maintained despite the Blackwell and Shepherd article, the situation in England and America was quite different – there, many clinicians were persuaded that the evidence for lithium prophylaxis was suspect, and lithium treatment was therefore suspended whilst the psychiatrists waited for the next round in the contest.

This was how matters stood in the summer of 1969. We found the evidence for a prophylactic action of lithium weighty; the Maudsley psychiatrists found it unconvincing. The controversy did not fail to affect the usage of lithium, and it did so differently in different parts of the world. In Scandinavia and Continental Europe lithium was being used increasingly and with good results. In England and America some psychiatrists took up the treatment and obtained the same good results, but other psychiatrists hesitated. They were impressed on the one side by the scientific debate, which seemed to leave much room for doubt about the efficacy of lithium, and on the other by the extra trouble and responsibility of lithium treatment.[45]

Baastrup and Schou felt that, in a way, they were partly responsible for this situation having arisen in the first place: had they done a double-blind trial before publicising their findings, there might never have arisen the degree of doubt about lithium prophylaxis which so affected prescribing practice in England and the USA. The Danes accepted this responsibility and it was a factor which argued in favour of a new clinical trial with double-blind and placebo controls – but was the argument strong enough?

Could we ... expose a random sample of our patients to placebo ... to painful relapses and possibly suicide in order to obtain evidence for the benefit of patients in England and the United States? To do so would presumably be against the Helsinki Declaration which clearly states that patients must not be exposed to risk through experiments unless these are of potential benefit to themselves.[46]

It was not possible to allow the responsibility to rest with the Maudsley psychiatrists since, as far as Baastrup and Schou could tell, all the indications were that they had no intention of planning and carrying out a trial of lithium. In the end, Baastrup and Schou decided to go ahead and to perform the necessary definitive trial but they did so only after they had designed a trial protocol which went some way to alleviating their ethical misgivings. The results of the study appeared in the *Lancet* of 15 August[47] in an article co-authored by Drs J. C. Poulsen, K. Thomsen and A. Amdisen. Schou has succinctly outlined the essential features of the study.[48]

> In this study eighty-four patients who had been in lithium treatment for a year or longer were switched double-blind to continued treatment with either lithium or placebo, the two treatments being allocated randomly. A sequential analysis design, pairing lithium-treated patients with placebo-treated patients, served to terminate the trial as soon as statistical significance ($p < 0.01$) had been achieved. During the trial, when a relapse occurred, the trial was terminated for that member of the pair, and treatment was immediately instituted to reverse the relapse. In this way, the numbers of relapses occurring, and of patients put at risk of relapse, were minimised, as were the ethical problems involved in withdrawing putatively effective treatment from patients apparently receiving benefit.
>
> The trial was terminated by the sequential design within six months, and the findings appeared unequivocal. At that time more than half of the patients given placebo had relapsed; none of the lithium patients had done so. In the view of the authors of the report, the prophylactic efficacy of lithium had been conclusively demonstrated.

Blackwell was not to be mollified, and wrote to the *Lancet*[49] to complain that the new clinical trial still possessed methodological inadequacies rendering the evidence unreliable. Specifically, he suggested that the placebo-treated patients might have been aware of the fact that their medication had been removed, particularly if previously noticeable lithium-induced side effects ceased to occur. The knowledge that they were not receiving medication might have alarmed the patients and hence precipitated relapse.

Mogens Schou replied[50] that all this was, of course, quite possible, but in view of the fact that no patient ever mentioned or reported the kind of effects required by Blackwell's explanation, it seemed most unlikely.

In fact, the double-blind discontinuation study virtually settled the prophylaxis issue. There were one or two rumblings[51] in the pages of the *Lancet* concerning the validity of the type of sequential trial design which had been used, but these came to nothing in the end.

Blackwell, however, still refused to be convinced. In 1972, in the *American Heart Journal*,[52] he continued to refer to 'the need for an adequate evaluation of this claim for prophylaxis'.[53] Even now he remains unrepentant:

> I believe that we were right to make the methodologic points that we did and that they were (and remain) valid. We were also wrong. I think that the weight of clinical conviction by this date is convincing and that lithium has a place in the prevention of manic relapses.
>
> However, I also think that the whole area of 'prophylaxis' and maintenance therapy should be very closely examined. The difference between dependency and prophylaxis may exist largely in the eye of the prescriber! I suspect that what has changed is not the weight of *scientific* evidence so much as the sheer *clinical* consensus concerning efficacy. If one were to submit current data to equally rigorous scrutiny it might still fall short of 'proof'.[54]

The one aspect of the whole controversy which produced the greatest frustration in the Danish psychiatrists was the apparent inability of their English counterparts to acknowledge that there had ever been any ethical dilemma prior to setting up the double-blind discontinuation trial. For Shepherd, the issue was a simple one: the evidence for lithium prophylaxis was inadequate and the treatment therefore of unproven efficacy. In 1974 he made his position plain:

> The problem created by Professor Schou was of his own making: he appears to have believed so firmly in his own judgement as to have concluded that independent assessment was unnecessary. The evidence which he presented was certainly incomplete ... and the history of physical treatment in psychiatry has unfortunately demonstrated too often the folly of relying on uncontrolled studies alone, however eminent and enthusiastic the clinical observers.... For this reason I am personally very glad that Professor Schou eventually felt able to overcome his scruples and to accept the widely accepted ethos of the scientific community.[55]

Shepherd added that there was an 'ethical need to stabilise the climate of medical and lay opinion which has been so perturbed by the extravagance of the claims advanced by proponents of lithium as a "prophylactic" agent'.[56]

Schou felt this view to be one-sided, arguing that ethical problems involved in placebo-controlled trials must depend on the investigator's own assessment of existing evidence. Even though Shepherd, who doubted the existing evidence concerning lithium prophylaxis, did not see any ethical problems in a controlled trial (but also did not carry out such a trial), a problem did inevitably exist for Baastrup and Schou, who found the existing evidence weighty as shown in their detailed response [57] to Blackwell and Shepherd's original critique.[58] Schou replied:

> Professor Shepherd shows grave concern for the perturbed climate of medical and lay opinion about lithium prophylaxis. Perhaps there would have been less perturbation if our Maudsley colleagues had been less dogmatically unwilling to admit evidence, any evidence, supporting the notion of a prophylactic lithium action.[59]

The *Lancet* and the *British Medical Journal*

There is also a curious side issue to the controversy which is worth remarking. The two major medical periodicals in the UK, the *Lancet* and the *British Medical Journal*, appeared to take opposing sides in the dispute. The *Lancet*, which had published the original article by Blackwell and Shepherd, carried an editorial in April 1969[60] in which the therapeutic myth arguments were repeated in all essentials, and which made particular reference to the criticism that the criteria for choosing patients in the Baastrup and Schou study might have led to an artefactual result when lithium therapy was introduced: to select patients having a recent history of frequent episodes might, the *Lancet* editorial suggested, be to select just those patients in whom there was likely to be a good prognosis. When the Danish psychiatrists submitted the manuscript of their double-blind discontinuation study to the *Lancet* they accompanied it with a second paper which addressed itself specifically to the issue of patient selection and presented data and calculations showing that the criteria adopted in the original work did not lead to the differential choice of good prognosis subjects. The editor of the *Lancet* rejected both articles, eventually agreeing to publish the double-blind discontinuation study only after the intervention of Professor Linford Rees who made a special appeal on behalf of Baastrup and Schou.[61] The second article was not accepted, however, even though it answered unequivocally one of the most crucial objections to the idea of lithium prophylaxis. It eventually appeared in *International Phamacopsychiatry*.[62]

Schou felt[63] the decision of the *Lancet* not to publish this crucial paper when the criticisms with which it dealt had appeared in the *Lancet*'s pages, was wrong. Moreover, he notes that no proofs were ever sent to him of the double-blind discontinuation study article, and when it finally appeared in print a proof-reading oversight[64] by the *Lancet*'s editorial staff had led to a crucial significance level of $p < 0.01$ appearing as $p < 0.1$.

The *British Medical Journal*, on the other hand, adopted a stance considerably more favourable to lithium. On 2 November 1968,[65] an editorial quoted approvingly the work of Jules Angst and his colleagues, and two years later a follow-up editorial[66] reaffirmed this position. Queries on lithium therapy directed to the 'Any Questions' columns of the *British*

Medical Journal[67] drew replies which did not express doubts as to the treatment's effectiveness.

At least one person was not affected by the apparent antipathetic attitude of the *Lancet*; John Cade, writing to Mogens Schou after the appearance of the double-blind discontinuation study article, thanked him for 'the copy of your memorable paper that was published (so reluctantly) by the *Lancet* recently',[68] and continued in characteristic style:

> They did not have the decency to produce an editorial annotation acknowledging that you and Poul had K-Oed Blackwell and Shepherd in the final round! No matter. Your contention has been proven so convincingly that the whole world must be persuaded.[69]

The importance of the 'therapeutic myth' debate

It is difficult to know what to make of this phase in the history of lithium therapy. At the time, the 'therapeutic myth controversy' aroused unpleasant emotions. No matter how fine the filter provided by the linguistic conventions of scientific communication, the personal feelings nevertheless came through and some appear to linger. In 1980 an unsigned review appeared in the journal edited by Michael Shepherd[70] of a book edited by Mogens Schou and Erik Strömgren.[71] The reviewer wrote:

> The most striking feature of the volume ... is the devotion of the first third of the contents to lithium and its clinical effects. The editors' explanation of this choice – that it reflects the usual sequence of events in clinical psychiatry – is somewhat ingenuous: the explosion of interest in lithium during the 1970s can be attributed in large measure to the Danish engineroom at Risskov and, in particular, to the tireless activity of Dr Mogens Schou. The essence of the story is contained in the first two chapters, both by Schou ... Now that the lithium bubble is bursting, such information may prove to be of some value to the future student of the natural history of overvalued treatments in psychiatry.[72]

Some of the participants in the controversy, however, remained generous in their assessment. Nathan Kline commented that, 'The exchange with Barry Blackwell, to the best of my recollection, was done in good humor and certainly did not involve any personal animus'.[73]

One may hope that the residuum of the therapeutic myth controversy may at last subside, since a recent report by the Medical Research Council Drug Trials Subcommittee[74] clearly established the prophylactic effect of lithium; Shepherd was a member of the Drug Trials Subcommittee and was responsible, with others, for preparing the report.

That important methodological issues were at stake during the 'therapeutic myth' debate is undeniable, and the force with which the arguments were repeated undoubtedly had a marked effect upon the degree of attention paid to the methodological issues in the conduct of clinical trials, not just in lithium research but in studies of other drugs too.[75] In trying to analyse why opinions became so divided, Schou wrote in 1973:

> To the nonpsychiatric bystander it must have caused astonishment that views so much in contrast to each other could be held by reputable psychiatrists. Even in the profession the debate generated concern, because it revealed a lack of solid knowledge about fundamental aspects of a supposedly well-known psychiatric disorder. It is presumably no coincidence that the protagonists in the debate were, respectively, psychiatrists of the Kraepelinian school with its emphasis on manic–depressive disorder as one of the endogenous psychoses, and psychiatrists trained in the school of Aubrey Lewis, where stress is laid on the clinical continuity between depressions precipitated by a clear-cut external event and depressions where such an event is less obvious but may still be suspected. The latter group of psychiatrists is more likely than the former to give strong weight to psychological factors and placebo controls. The debate served to highlight important unanswered questions.[76]

Schou has later provided the following comment:

> In my lectures on psychiatric pharmacotherapy for medical students I use the historical development of lithium treatment to illustrate methodological and ethical issues involved in the testing and documentation of drug effects. It would hardly be possible for me to disguise my personal involvement in the matter, and I make no attempt at doing this, but the lecture concludes with the following re-establishment of proportions: 'My presentation may have led you to see this scientific controversy as a kind of fight or game in which the participants tried to score over each other, and that is to some extent also how it was felt at the time. Baastrup and I disliked the arguments *ad hominen* that were taken in use by our critics. But you must understand that we did – and do – welcome criticism that deals with substance, with data and their interpretation. Scientific research can flourish only in critical dialogue, and as far as lithium prophylaxis is concerned there is no doubt that the valid parts of the criticism had a positive effect by promoting further testing and thus indirectly providing still more solid documentation.'[77]

In retrospect, the years 1968 to 1970 remain as a disquieting interlude in the lithium story. It is particularly remarkable for the occasionally intemperate language employed in certain of the articles and the depth of feeling displayed. Shepherd and Blackwell undoubtedly had an important point to make, but the manner of making it produced effects other than those which, in a purely scientific sense, were desirable. The intensity of the controversy might well have forced the participants into entrenched positions from which any movement would have been difficult, but Baastrup and Schou did respond by performing their double-blind trial. Lithium therapy is not, however, the only area of clinical research ever to have seen controversy which has drawn individuals into personal arguments, and perhaps one should not, for that reason, make too much of it in this case.

8
The spread of lithium therapy

In recent times, the advent of computerised systems for information storage, classification, retrieval and dissemination has made the communication of scientific ideas a very rapid and generalised process. It is no longer possible to trace, with any degree of precision, who told what to whom, when, and with what effect. To the historian interested in disentangling the social from the scientific elements in the spread of ideas, this communications revolution has been a disaster of immense proportions.

When John Cade made his discovery, however, ideas were still dependent for their dissemination on the chance reading of an article by a few interested individuals who would then pass on the ideas by word of mouth to their colleagues. The database had yet to supercede the lunchtime chat over a drink.

It is, therefore, to some extent possible to determine how lithium therapy came to be adopted in the United Kingdom, the USA, and other countries around the world, though some uncertainties remain. The story may be read at many levels. It may be viewed simply as the operation of a fairly inefficient and idiosyncratic communications network, or it may be taken as illustrating how a few individuals whose receptiveness to new ideas was above the average, seized upon a promising suggestion and by experiment, astute observation, and not a little guesswork and faith, amplified the weak signal into a loud and clear message which others could not ignore.

The spread of lithium owed much to individuals who just happened to be in the right place at the right time and who had not only the perspicacity to recognise a bright idea when they saw one but the enthusiasm to pursue it.

The United States of America

There are four possible routes by which the idea of lithium therapy could, in principle, have entered the USA – directly from Australia; from Denmark, from the United Kingdom or from some other country. In fact, the available evidence seems to point to only the first two of these actually having been involved to any important extent.

The Australian connection is particularly clear in the influence which Samuel Gershon[1] had upon a number of American clinicians and research workers.

Gershon had worked with Trautner at the University of Melbourne, and had played a leading role in a number of interesting and well-designed investigations dealing with various practical aspects of lithium treatment and lithium toxicity. In 1959 and 1960, whilst spending a year as an Associate in Psychiatry at the University of Michigan, he collaborated with Arthur Yuwiler on the preparation of what was to be the first US publication on clinical lithium studies[2] reviewing what was known up to that time about the therapeutic effectiveness of lithium in affective disorders and a number of other conditions, as well as the more important therapeutic procedures. This article was certainly influential in alerting American psychiatrists to the existence of lithium therapy at a time when the Australian and Danish studies were scarcely known in the USA.

It was three years after the appearance of this paper, in 1963, that Gershon moved to the United States to take up the first of a series of senior positions in university departments of psychiatry and various clinical institutes in that country. It was from this time that his interest in lithium therapy really started to transmit itself to others.

Sam Gershon is an energetic, friendly and witty individual with an infectious enthusiasm for his work: a number of investigators have no difficulty in tracing their own involvement with lithium therapy to his influence. For example, Robert Prien,[3] a Research Psychologist with the National Institute of Mental Health, records that he became interested in lithium therapy in 1966 when he joined the planning committee for a multi-hospital study sponsored jointly by the Veterans' Administration and the National Institute of Mental Health (VA-NIMH); at this time, Prien was grateful to be able to draw upon Gershon's advice and expertise: the subsequent collaboration which Prien had with Gershon in planning research projects and preparing papers was rated by Prien as one of the major influences on his work.

Joyce Small[4] of Indianapolis, who has long been in the forefront of research on electroencephalographic effects of lithium and who has, in addition, made notable contributions to many other aspects of lithium therapy, had her interest in the subject first stimulated around 1959 when she and Gershon were in Michigan. She subsequently collaborated with Robert Prien in the VA-NIMH study.

Andrew Ho,[5] Associate Professor of Pharmacology at Peoria School of Medicine, became interested in lithium as a graduate student at Melbourne University between 1963 and 1967, and then carried out research into lithium effects on brain biogenic amines and electrolytes, working with

Gershon at the New York University Medical Center which Gershon had joined in 1965 as Research Associate Professor of Psychiatry (becoming Professor of Psychiatry in 1971).

The Danish work on lithium came to America through Dr Heinrich Waelsch, Chief Biochemist at the New York State Psychiatric Institute. Mogens Schou had earlier spent a year working with Waelsch, and the two had discussed the whole issue of lithium therapy. Subsequently, Waelsch maintained his interest in the topic, keeping abreast of the literature on it, and in 1958 he talked about his interest in lithium to a medical resident at the Psychiatric Institute, by the name of Ronald Fieve. At about the same time, Dr Lawrence Kolb, then Director of the Institute also raised the matter with Ron Fieve. Kolb was very familiar with the details of the early Danish and Australian lithium trials, having attended conferences in both countries where the trials had been reported. Fieve's interest was immediately aroused by the new treatment and, under Kolb's encouragement, he started lithium treatment in a number of manic–depressive patients who had failed to respond to other forms of medication. According to Fieve,[6] these constituted the earliest trials at the Institute (around the end of 1958 and into 1959 and 1960) and were probably the first systematic trials of lithium in the USA conducted by any American psychiatrist.

It was, however, a Canadian, rather than an American, who published the first North American report of a successful clinical trial of lithium; this was Edward Kingstone of the Allan Memorial Institute of Psychiatry in Montreal. Whilst this might properly be considered a Canadian development, the results of Kingstone's open trial of seventeen manic patients appeared in *Comprehensive Psychiatry*, an American journal read widely in the United States.[7] Nevertheless, Kingstone had little further influence upon the establishment of lithium therapy in the USA.

Fieve, however, pursued the matter with considerable vigour. He conducted open and single-blind trials of lithium in the late 1950s and early 1960s, going on to develop an entire department of lithium studies in manic–depressive disorders at the New York State Psychiatric Institute and Columbia Presbyterian Medical Center, which he has continued to head since 1962.

Early in the 1960s, Fieve set up the first 'lithium clinic', a term which he himself coined. Later, in 1975, he established the first Lithium Foundation for Depression and Manic–Depression in New York City.

It was in 1975 that *Moodswing*[8] appeared: this was a book which Fieve had written to present, to a wide general public, the lithium story as seen from his own vantage point as a clinician and scientist. The book was an astounding success, becoming so popular throughout the United States that hundreds of thousands of copies were sold: by 1980 it had been translated into four other languages and had sold in excess of one million copies in the English edition alone.

Fieve's path, as he himself describes it, was not, however, always an easy one. After opening the lithium clinic in New York City, he made a proposal to the Commissioner of Mental Health in New York State that similar clinics should be developed and set up in all of the major New York State mental hospitals. There was, according to Fieve, immediate opposition to this idea. Nathan Kline, who had introduced antidepressants into the New York State system, convened an all-day discussion session on the topic, bringing in a number of others who were opposed to Fieve's idea of state lithium clinics. The proposal was allowed to lapse until, about two years later, Fieve put it to the National Institute of Health. Whilst indicating interest, the NIH turned the matter over to the National Institute of Mental Health which in turn referred it to Dr Jerome Levine who headed the Psychopharmacology Branch. Again, a full day's meeting was convened of psychopharmacologists and experts on lithium therapy. The majority voted against the provision of federal funds to support lithium clinics throughout the country. At the time Ron Fieve felt the defeat keenly, believing as he did that in the long term the lithium clinics which he had proposed would more than justify the expenditure involved in their establishment by reducing the costs of repeated hospitalisation resulting from recurrent affective disorders. It is with some personal satisfaction that Fieve is at the present time able to point to what he sees as the vindication of his position:

> Ironically, despite the strong opposition of my state and federal colleagues, the final outcome ... is that lithium clinics have proliferated throughout New York State and in most of the major university teaching hospitals across the United States. The term 'lithium clinic' has prevailed, although in some instances they have been called affective disorder clinics, or depression clinics, and in one case 'mood clinic'.[9]

Of course, the way in which events are perceived, interpreted and remembered depends very much upon the role which an individual plays in them, and Fieve's picture of the opposition which he encountered is not shared by others. Samuel Gershon, for example, comments:

> To my knowledge there was no meeting at which the positive or negative features were discussed in a public forum which would have any impact on anybody's decision and secondly, [the] so-called affective disorders clinics or lithium clinics had been set up in Australia and they were in fact set up at New York University when I came there. Therefore, this whole issue about an opposition to the proposal presented by Fieve seems to me unclear and unconfirmed.[10]

Ron Fieve has never been one to shun the full glare of publicity and has, indeed, often appeared to seek a public platform for his opinions. This is consistent with his view that the better education of the man in the street concerning the nature of mood disorders and the availability of effective treatment techniques, may be a powerful force in adjusting attitudes towards depression and manic–depression and in helping to reduce the misunderstanding and prejudice which surrounds such conditions. In the early 1970s, this was illustrated in a particularly dramatic way. Joshua Logan, the American playwright, producer and director (of *South Pacific* and *Camelot*, for example) was one of Fieve's patients: Logan's manic–depression had been brought under control with lithium, and he and Fieve had been interviewed by major television networks and newspapers. In 1973, Fieve invited Logan to take part in a panel discussion organised by the American Medical Association and televised nationwide. Fieve and Logan were interviewed by fifty members of the American press and television on the furore surrounding the affair of Senator Tom Eagleton, Vice Presidential running mate of Senator McGovern in the Presidential election campaign which was then in full swing. Senator Eagleton, a pleasant, good-looking, personable individual, was nevertheless revealed to have suffered in the past from recurrent episodes of depression for which he had received treatment, and he was consequently forced to drop out of the campaign. Liberal opinion was scandalised by the destruction of a political career for such a reason, and public interest in the television programme was enormous; in Fieve's view it helped to generate a widespread acceptance of lithium therapy in the United States at a crucial time for the establishment of psychiatric treatment services.[11]

It is not only in the public domain that Fieve's influence has been felt. In 1970 the task force set up by the Food and Drug Administration in conjunction with the American Psychiatric Association to look into the lithium question, included Fieve as one of its members, and he has continued to be a major voice in the task force's pronouncements on lithium ever since. Fieve recounts how his successful treatment of manic–depression using lithium so impressed certain other psychiatrists that they too started to investigate the new therapy:

> Early in the 1960s Schlagenhauf and Tupin called me from Texas and asked that I hospitalise a manic professor who had written 20 books and 50 papers and who was uncontrolled in a state Texas mental hospital on massive doses of thorazine. To date they had never used lithium but had heard that I was using lithium at New York State Psychiatric Institute and they wanted to send him up for a trial. When the Texas professor arrived, he was wild, elated and not sleeping at all. After 7–8 weeks of lithium therapy he calmed down to a normal-thymic state and he was shipped back to Texas. Thereafter Schlagenhauf, White, Tupin and their associates began similar trials of lithium in manic states such as the ones we had been conducting openly but had not yet published at the New York State Psychiatric Institute. In 1965–66 both the Schlagenhauf series[12] and my series[13] . . . were published.[14]

Joe Tupin[15] himself saw this as a turning point in his investigations:

> My first interest in lithium was stimulated by seeing a patient who was on lithium and doing well after a long history of serious cyclic affective disturbance. This was in 1964. The patient had been seen by the group at Columbia University, New York City.[16]

At the time, Tupin was working with two colleagues, Robert B. White and George Schlagenhauf, at the University of Texas,Galveston. After seeing the dramatic effects of lithium on the one patient, Tupin decided to set up an open clinical study and applied to the FDA for the necessary forms to file for permission to investigate lithium; permission was granted, and Tupin became the first person in the USA to obtain an IND (permission to investigate a new drug) for lithium. He recalls the circumstances surrounding the IND application:

> Various questions were asked and I answered most from the existing literature drawing from work in other countries including that done by Schou, Gershon and Cade. One question that was asked was the chemical composition and purity of the lithium which was to be used. Since none was available, I obtained a reagent grade bulk lithium carbonate, prepared for laboratory purposes. . . . I transferred the assay information on the label of that lithium carbonate to the application, verbatim, and that became the basis for the first official approval in this country.[17]

The results of the study were reported at the American Psychiatric Association meeting in New York City in the spring of 1966, the same meeting at which Fieve reported his findings, and subsequently appeared later that same year in the *American Journal of Psychiatry*.[18]

In spite of the efforts of those who, like Gershon, Tupin and Fieve, publicised and promoted further investigations into the therapeutic effects of lithium, there was a background of mistrust of lithium to be overcome in the United States – mistrust and often downright ignorance. American psychiatrists, looking for guidance on the topic in the well-respected 1956 second edition of *The Pharmacological Basis of Therapeutics* edited by L. S. Goodman and A. Gilman[19] would read:

> The lithium ion has no therapeutic applications and, so far as is known, no biological function. Indeed, the only pharmacological interest in lithium arises from the fact that the ion is toxic. Even this would be only of academic interest were it not for the fact that lithium salts have been employed as flavoring agents in low-sodium diets and have caused poisoning.[20]

In answer to a question to the editor of the *Journal of the American Medical Association* as to whether there was any legitimate medical use for the compounds of lithium, Dr Christian Wingard (described in an editorial footnote as a 'competent authority') declared, 'There are no therapeutic uses for lithium salts':[21] this was in 1961!

Bob Prien recalls the atmosphere of scepticism which surrounded clinical research on lithium at that time:

> There was significant resistance to lithium therapy in the United States when we were planning the first major collaborative study in the mid-1960s. Up to that time there had been some isolated small sample research by groups in New York and Texas but nothing that had caught on in the field. When the possibility of a government-sponsored lithium project was first considered in 1965, there was a widespread reaction of amusement followed by astonishment when it was realised that we were actually serious about the project. The spectre of the calamities with lithium chloride as a salt substitute in 1949 was still fresh in the minds of many clinicians. Very few clinicians had heard of Schou or any of the work done with lithium in Europe and Australia. One prominent research scientist asked me when we were considering reviving psychosurgery. It was difficult recruiting treatment centers for the project and even more difficult in persuading many of the participating clinicians that they were not dealing with an extremely unsafe treatment. Once the study had progressed for a few years, the attitude of the participating clinicians changed drastically and many were then seriously concerned about administering a placebo when an effective treatment such as lithium was available.[22]

The 'spectre of the calamities' of 1949, to which Prien referred was not so easily expunged from official consciousness, however. The Food and Drug Administration, having had its fingers badly burnt on one occasion, was not particularly enthusiastic about giving the go-ahead for the use of lithium compounds in clinical psychiatry, and for as long as ten years following the appearance of the articles by Gershon and Yuwiler[23] and Kingstone[24] the FDA did not permit lithium to be marketed for use on general prescription.

As the evidence for clinical efficacy mounted, however, so the pressure grew on the FDA to liberalise its position on lithium, and several prominent psychiatrists made public pleas that this should happen. One such was Jonathon Cole;[25] writing in the editorial columns of the *American Journal of Psychiatry* in October 1968,[26] he drew attention to the fact that 'without the encouragement of sponsorship by any commercial drug firm, more than 200 psychiatrists have applied individually to the Food and Drug Administration for permission to study and use this compound as a treatment for affective disorders',[27] and he noted that the clinical effectiveness of lithium was felt to be so well established to the satisfaction of a large number of psychiatrists that in many cases the drug was being employed without FDA permission, the tablets being obtained from various sources.

Cole's appeal was a strong one, and is worth recording in some detail:

The FDA has been quite helpful to clinicians wishing to file Investigation-al New Drug (IND) requests for permission to study lithium clinically. However, a number of investigators feel that the available evidence is already adequate to permit the drug to be marketed for general prescrip-tion use; they believe that this would have happened some time ago if some person or group had a financial interest in this inexpensive and unpatentable medication.

My appraisal of the existing situation is as follows:

1. There is ample evidence that lithium carbonate, used with proper clinical and laboratory precautions, is a safe and effective treatment for acute mania.

2. It is less clear as to whether lithium is a better or faster treatment for manic states than the phenothiazines or haloperidol.

3. There is reasonable but not overwhelming evidence that the drug, administered for months and years, may avert future attacks of either depression or mania in patients with recurrent affective illnesses of either or both types. . . .

The question then is: 'Given an intriguing and unique drug treatment with demonstrated efficacy in a limited condition, mania, and great promise in a much more important clinical area, the prevention of serious affective illnesses, what should a regulatory agency do?'[28]

Cole put forward a number of suggestions for ways in which the FDA might proceed. There were two proposals in particular which were of considerable importance:

Approval of an effective New Drug Application for the use of lithium in manic states should be expedited by the FDA. The APA and perhaps other agencies should work with the FDA, if invited, to help develop appropriate labeling for safe use.[29]

Central single sponsorship of uncontrolled single-blind clinical studies of lithium as a preventive treatment should be developed to relieve indi-vidual investigators of the problem of sponsoring INDs if they agree to collect systematic standard data on their patients as part of a larger program.

This last recommendation would help avert the rapidly spreading informal use of the drug, allow rapid communication of new knowledge about lithium, and facilitate the eventual approval of the prescription use of lithium as a prophylactic therapy. . . .

The major alternative would be the approval of the prophylactic use of lithium carbonate under carefully specified conditions as part of the labeling under the New Drug Application noted above . . . I believe that the world experience with this drug is sufficient to make it likely that benefits of such broadened use would outweigh the hazards.[30]

Nathan Kline recalls[31] that the FDA was eventually so inundated with applications from psychiatrists for permission to carry out supposed investigations of lithium (in fact, of course, they wished merely to use it to treat patients) that many of the FDA staff were eager to grant the approval simply to avoid having to process further applications. Kline himself had been active in campaigning for lithium; together with a group of other interested clinicians he engaged in discussions with the FDA. At one time, the American College of Neuropsychopharmacology, of which Kline was an active member, seriously considered putting in a New Drug Application on its own behalf in order to get lithium released for general prescription, and only decided not to do so when it was learned that applications were already being made by three pharmaceutical companies.

At about the same time that Cole, Kline, and a number of others were putting their case to the FDA, Smith, Kline and French, J. B. Roerig Division of Pfizer Inc, and Rowell Laboratories Inc, had been engaged in preliminary investigations of lithium, and virtually simultaneously submitted New Drug Applications to the FDA in respect of lithium carbonate. As Cole noted,[32] this action relieved the FDA of the need to take the initiative and one and a half years later, on 6 April 1970, the FDA issued an information sheet[33] announcing that all three applications had been approved. As from 1 June that year, three lithium carbonate preparations were to be made available[34] – Eskalith®, Lithonate® and Lithane®, the first two being capsules and the last a scored tablet.

There was, however, a catch. Despite Cole's suggestion that the evidence for a prophylactic use of lithium against recurrent affective episodes was sufficiently encouraging to warrant the drug being prescribed for such a purpose, the FDA did not agree.

> The sole indication for the use of lithium carbonate at this time is for control of manic episodes of manic psychosis. Evidence for efficacy in other indications is not yet available.[35]

> The value of lithium carbonate in preventing or lessening the frequency or severity of manic episodes is the subject of continuing investigation with findings thus far inconclusive.[36]

The role of lithium in the prophylactic treatment of recurrent depression was not even mentioned. This limited approval of lithium remained the FDA's position until 1974 when a decision was made to approve the use of lithium for the prophylactic treatment of bipolar affective illness, but the approval for unipolar recurrent depression was – and still is – withheld. The 1974 decision of the FDA was based primarily upon data gathered in an eighteen-hospital Veterans' Administration and National Institute of Mental Health collaborative study conducted under the supervision of Bob Prien.[37]

There are those, particularly in the UK and continental Europe but also in the USA, who feel that the conservative approach consistently adopted by the FDA is quite unjustified. Jonathon Himmelhoch,[38] for example, believes that the FDA has always treated psychiatric medication over-cautiously:

> In the US, psychiatric therapies, lithium included, have always been judged according to special guidelines. Methyltrexate was released to treat psoriasis, but the FDA took 21 years to release lithium. The only conclusion one can deduce from this is that the operating hypothesis of the FDA . . . is that . . . mental illness is not 'real' but the patients' own damn fault – therefore drugs for such folly must have a zero-to-infinity risk-benefit ratio. 'Real' diseases, from psoriasis to cancer, can be treated with any poison, triple therapies abound, and organ transplants are the cat's pajamas.[39]

Others, however, are of the opinion that the FDA was, and is, right to adopt the conservative approach; Peter Stokes[40] put it like this:

> I must say that the action of governmental agencies as regards lithium use in the United states has been reasonable and informed. It has persuaded the scientific community that we should proceed from the vantage of reasonable, thoughtful and *researched* viewpoints. I happen to subscribe to the general precept that first of all we as physicians 'should do no harm'. This places us necessarily in a conservative approach to new therapies.[41]

Joe Tupin concurs:

> Generally, in this country, I believe that government agencies have been rather flexible, forward looking, and helpful in advancing lithium.[42]

Sam Gershon, one of the members of the APA task force on lithium has similar views:

> Currently the FDA has a conservative approach to [lithium] use and indications but overall this seems not inappropriate to the total data base given the various areas of current controversy.[43]

Bob Prien, another task force member, also thinks that the FDA stance has much to recommend it:

> I . . . feel that the Food and Drug Administration has been judicious in [its] decisions regarding approval of lithium therapy. I disagree with some

of my colleagues who feel that the FDA has been remiss in not approving
the use of lithium for the long-term maintenance treatment of unipolar
recurrent affective illness.[44]

Despite these endorsements of FDA policy, it remains true that the USA
is out of line with most other countries as far as the officially sanctioned uses
of lithium are concerned and while it is difficult to avoid the conclusion that
this is to a large extent a legacy of the lithium toxicity debacle of 1949, it
would be unfair to suggest that this is the only reason. There can, however,
be no doubt that official reluctance to embrace lithium therapy had an effect
upon its general acceptance by the medical profession and upon the acquisi-
tion of clinical experience of its use. It did, of course, also mean that patients
who might have benefited from lithium were, in many cases, denied access to
the treatment. In the words of Jonathon Himmelhoch:

> The slow acceptance of lithium therapy was a national embarassment. If
> one could multiply individual morbidity from bipolar illness by the
> number of years it took for treatment to reach a suffering population, the
> figure would be a tragic one.... In recent years we have been doing
> better, and have not suffered greatly from controls.... True, lithium is
> still not approved for many situations, including depressive episodes,
> where it can be effective. But, on the other hand, everybody ignores these
> restraints.[45]

Lithium research, both clinical and laboratory-based, has been carried out
in the United States on a scale unequalled in any other country. It is, in many
ways, invidious even to attempt to distinguish the contributions made by
only four or five investigators when the free-ranging scientific contacts for
which the USA is justly renowned make it certain that the lines of communication, encouragement and influence must have been very complex indeed,
involving individuals whose vital roles are doomed to remain in obscurity –
unrecognised and unapplauded.

The United Kingdom

To the British, Australia has never been quite the remote and little-known
place which it often seems to the Americans or continental Europeans.
Once a possession of the Empire and now a major partner in the Common-
wealth, Australia has strong cultural and academic links with Britain, and
Australian medical journals are held by virtually all medical school libraries
in Britain and are widely consulted. It seems likely, therefore, that the news
of the possible therapeutic effectiveness of lithium spread to Britain as a
direct result of the appearance in print of the work of John Cade and of
Edward Trautner and his colleagues.

The first British publication on lithium appeared in the *Journal of Mental Science* in 1956,[46] its author being Dr David Rice, a consultant psychiatrist and at that time Deputy Medical Superintendent of Graylingwell Hospital in Chichester, England. Rice's article was brief, and recorded the outcome of lithium treatment in twenty-seven male and thirty-one female patients: he concluded that lithium was an effective treatment of mania and hypomania and that where improvement occurred in patients of mixed symptomatology this was due to an alleviation of the affective element.

Rice has given a little of the background to his work:[47]

It all occurred almost by default, or accident. It was in about 1952–53 when I was in charge of the male side at Graylingwell Hospital, Chichester. I had at that time two particularly difficult and overactive patients with long hypomanic (manic) illnesses. In those days our pharmacological armamentarium was pretty limited.... I would have liked to give each of these chaps ECT but the relatives wouldn't allow it. We were pondering on what we could do when an Australian Registrar[48] produced a scruffy crumpled sheet from the journal of the Australian Medical Association[49] with Cade's article in it.[50] I felt we had nothing to lose so decided to try it.

Rice originally wrote up the details of the treatment for a research prize awarded by the Regional Hospital Board. It was not successful. The manuscript was then submitted for publication. In the early stages of the study, after the first two patients did well, Rice discussed the results with the medical staff at Graylingwell and thereafter all potentially suitable patients were referred to him for lithium treatment enabling him to collect the fifty-eight patients for his study.

In 1956, at about the time that his paper appeared in the *Journal of Mental Science*, Rice moved to Hellingly Hospital at Hailsham, Sussex, where he became a close colleague and friend of Dr Ronald Maggs, another consultant psychiatrist. Maggs' interest was immediately stimulated by Rice's account of his work and together they held frequent discussions about lithium therapy. Maggs recalls the time clearly:

David Rice ... had been impressed by ... news of John Cade's work which had been described at Graylingwell by an Australian Registrar or Senior Registrar whom I never heard mentioned by name, let alone met. . . . It followed quite naturally that upon Dr Rice moving eastwards along the coast to Hellingly he should tell us of the good news.... One of his Graylingwell patients appeared to be very similar to one of my disturbed patients and I thought it worthwhile to try the effect of lithium.... The results made such an impression upon me that in spite of the development of the phenothiazines and the many social changes that were taking place in psychiatry at the time ... I considered that this subject was worthy of further research.[51]

David Rice was not himself inclined to follow up his observations by a planned clinical trial ('I am afraid I haven't got a research mind'[52]) and was happy enough to leave this side of things to Ronald Maggs. Maggs made an application to the South-East Metropolitan Regional Health Committee for a grant so that he could collaborate with his colleagues in the Pathology Department of his hospital in setting up measurements of serum lithium levels during treatment in association with a double-blind clinical trial of lithium against mania. The results of this trial, which fully confirmed the clinical efficacy of lithium, were published in the *British Journal of Psychiatry* in 1963.[53]

Both Rice and Maggs knew Hartigan of St Augustine's, Canterbury; the stimulus for Hartigan's own work came from Rice.[54] Maggs met Hartigan only once, and that was after the publication of Hartigan's paper in 1963.

Maggs was acquainted with a psychiatrist from West Park Hospital, Epsom – Dr Alec Coppen. Coppen had been invited to Hellingly Hospital on several occasions to give scientific papers, and he and Maggs became involved in joint work on chemotherapeutic aspects of the affective disorders; they also shared a common interest in lithium therapy. Coppen was particularly intrigued by the possibility that lithium might be prophylactically effective against recurrent affective disturbances, including depressive relapses, and invited Maggs to take part in a large-scale multi-hospital trial which he was planning to look into the question. Maggs readily agreed, having already heard Schou speak on the matter at the International Congress of Psychiatry in 1966.[55]

> Although I felt that the paper that Schou and his colleagues gave in 1966 on prophylaxis left much to be desired from the scientific aspect, I perceived sufficient substance within it to justify an involvement in the prophylactic study.[56]

The clinical trial which Coppen had organised involved eight psychiatrists in four hospitals.[57] The design was elegant and avoided the ethical pitfalls which so exercised Baastrup and Schou. The patients were allocated to lithium or placebo treatment groups, the study was conducted double-blind, and patients were allowed to receive whatever other medication or treatment was deemed necessary to alleviate mood disturbance during the trial. The trial continued over a two-year period, at the end of which time the effectiveness of the lithium treatment was assessed on a number of parameters, including global ratings of psychiatric status, amount of affective illness occurring during the trial, and the extent to which other treatments had proved necessary: on all measures, lithium was found to have been much more effective than placebo. Both bipolar and unipolar conditions responded to lithium prophylaxis, and the findings were not susceptible to interpretation on the basis of observer bias or the breaking of the drug-placebo blind. The finding was all the more impressive since the patients in the placebo group were not untreated, but received ECT or other antimanic and antidepressant drugs as necessary, thereby biasing the trial against lithium.

The British prophylactic trial was planned well before the appearance of the *Lancet* article of Blackwell and Shepherd[58] and the controversy which that provoked. It is interesting to speculate that the Blackwell and Shepherd critique might never have been made – or at least might have been stated less forcefully – had the British trial been published earlier, since it did exactly what Blackwell and Shepherd argued that Baastrup and Schou ought to have done, namely to provide unequivocal evidence of the superiority of lithium over placebo in a double-blind controlled clinical trial. Certainly the British trial never came under serious critical fire from any source, and a number of investigators are clear that it was this work, rather than that of the Danes, which first convinced them of the seriousness of the claim that lithium had prophylactic efficacy against recurrent depression.

Other countries

The adoption of lithium therapy by countries other than Great Britain and the USA has been uneven. In Scandinavia, the acceptance of lithium as an effective agent for both acute and prophlyactic treatment of recurrent mood disorders was very rapid, with few dissenting voices, a fact which presumably may be traced to the pioneering work of the Danish investigators.

In Canada, there has been a tendency, not entirely unexpected, for the fortunes of lithium therapy to follow fairly closely the pattern of usage in the USA. It was mentioned earlier[59] that it was Edward Kingstone, a Canadian, who had published the first North American paper on lithium therapy.[60] At the First Canadian International Symposium on Lithium, held in Quebec in 1974, Kingstone described how it was that he first came to hear about lithium. He was a resident at the Allan Memorial Institute in Montreal, the Director being Dr D. Ewen Cameron.[61]

As I remember, during ward rounds one day in the latter part of 1959, the team was discussing the treatment of patients on one of the wards at the Institute. Ward rounds then consisted of the same routine, by and large, as ward rounds do these days. That is to say, a group of doctors, nurses and other staff sitting around in office, surrounded by charts going over the reports of the various staff interactions with a particular patient. During these rounds the service chief, who was Dr Cameron, with myself as the senior resident, would make suggestions or requests that would send us scurrying off to the literature which in effect usually opened up a completely new horizon of endeavour or thought about a particular problem. This day in question was no exception and during what seemed to be the usual discussion about the treatment and progress of a patient suffering from a manic disorder, Dr Cameron turned to me and suggested we try lithium on this patient. He casually mentioned that there was a reference in the *Journal of Mental Science* (now called the *British Journal of Psychiatry*). The reference was to the publication by Rice in 1956 about the treatment of some 58 patients in Great Britain. At first it seemed reasonable to assume that this would end nowhere – another wild idea – but always to improve our knowledge and capabilities. Having discovered an entrée into the literature on this subject and having received the commission to investigate the usefulness of this drug, I began to discover the other sources of knowledge on this subject that existed at that time.[62]

Kingstone's account is particularly interesting in that it illustrates clearly how the several problems facing any investigator taking an interest in lithium at that time were tackled and overcome:

Perhaps a word should also be said about the research climate concerning new drugs that existed at that time. The easiest way to put it in context is to mention that this was in the years before the thalidomide tragedies. At that time each investigator acted as his own 'ethics committee'. As there was no manufacturer distributing lithium carbonate for use in any specific condition, it was necessary to appeal to the hospital's pharmacy to obtain and put up the medication in usable form. As it turned out, this was not a difficult thing to do inasmuch as a biological grade of lithium carbonate was all that we needed and this was easily available. The pharmacy arranged with a small pharmaceutical manufacturer to put up the medication in usable form. As I remember, because of the small cost involved, the pharmacy was able to obtain it without charge. The biochemistry technicians at the Institute quickly set up a method for detecting lithium in the blood. We were then able to proceed.[63]

Kingstone's clinical results with lithium were promising and he had managed to avoid problems of toxicity by adjusting dose levels for each individual according to the clinical effects obtained. A decision was therefore taken to publish the findings.

The results were written up including some case histories to represent the variety of situations seen: that is, a case that responded, a case that did not respond and a case whose response was somewhat ambiguous. All of this was sent off to the *Journal of the American Psychiatric Association* whose editor at that time resided in Toronto. In short order a letter came back and (if I remember correctly) the words were to the effect that the data and contents of the article would not be of interest to the readers of the journal. This message was difficult to interpret. It was then decided to submit it to another journal which had just come on the scene, namely *Comprehensive Psychiatry*, of which Dr Cameron was an editor.[64]

What Kingstone goes on to say next is of considerable import.

[Dr Cameron] suggested that the cases should be those of our best successes and not to represent any failures. His interpretation was that the readership interpreted the case results with the understanding that the worst cases were probably not being reported.[65]

John Cade had also given[66] an optimistic picture of his results which was not, perhaps, entirely justified by the information which he had to hand about the toxic and side effects of lithium. It cannot be ruled out as a possibility that had Kingstone not angled his report, as Cameron had suggested, to underplay the less successful clinical results, the impact upon other psychiatrists would have been much less, and follow-up work retarded.

After the acceptance of his article for publication, Kingstone went for a period to the Maudsley Hospital in England where, he discovered, 'lithium carbonate was not being used and was not even being considered'.[67]

Lithium therapy continued to make advances in Australia and in western Europe. In Ireland in 1963 Professor Norman Moore, Medical Director of St Patrick's Hospital, Dublin, read the article by G. P. Hartigan[68] which had appeared in the *British Journal of Psychiatry* and called it to the attention of Dr Patrick Melia, a psychiatrist working at St Patrick's Hospital. Moore suggested that Melia should review the literature; this he did, and after a discussion at a meeting of medical staff it was decided that he should conduct a pilot trial of lithium as a prophylactic in recurrent affective disorders. This was started in 1964 and the early results of the trial were encouraging: Melia visited Dr Alec Coppen at Epsom, in England, to discuss them. The pilot study findings were published in 1967 in the *Journal of the Irish Medical Association*.[69] Coppen, who had been a former senior colleague of Melia, encouraged Melia to do a double-blind trial. Melia took the advice and began the trial at St Patrick's Hospital in 1966; a preliminary report appeared in 1968 in the *Lancet*,[70] the full report being published in the *British Journal of Psychiatry* two years later.[71] Melia's work was not only methodologically sound, but also well written, and must have added considerable authority to the growing evidence of the prophylactic effect of lithium.

Lithium therapy became widely known in Greece through the writings of Dr G. N. Christodolou,[72] and in Spain through the work and writings of Professor J. J. Lopez-Ibor Aliño.[73]

In Italy, Dr Athanasio Kukopulos and his group[74] were largely responsible for a resurgence of interest in lithium in that country. Very often the direct influence of Mogens Schou may be readily detected in these developments. Kukopulos, for example, traces his interest in lithium to a personal contact which he had with Schou:

In autumn 1969 I received a letter from the husband of a former patient of mine saying that his wife was taking lithium with good results. Having treated this patient in previous years and knowing the strong tendency of her affective disorder to recur, I immediately thought that lithium was very likely the cause of her improvement. I telephoned Dr Mogens Schou to ask for an appointment to discuss lithium prophylactic therapy. He agreed to meet me, and I went to Risskov in December 1969 and spent 3 days with him. Since then I have been using lithium in my work.[75]

In Israel lithium began to be used sporadically on an experimental basis in the late 1960s and early 1970s, often by psychiatrists who had recently migrated to Israel from countries where lithium therapy was quite widely used. Dr Elliot S. Gershon was one such immigrant. In 1968 he had been a clinical associate at the National Institute of Mental Health, working with Drs William E. Bunney, Jr and Fred Goodwin. During that time, Elliot Gershon also collaborated with Dr Joseph Schildkraut whose interest lay in the biogenic amines and their role in affective disorders, and it was through Schildkraut that Gershon first became acquainted with lithium research. When eventually he moved to Israel, where he became Director of Research at the Jerusalem Mental Health Centre, Gershon took with him his new-found interest in lithium and decided to look further into the issues of unipolar and bipolar differences in antidepressant responses to lithium. It was at this point that the difficulties began.

The hospital was very supportive, but I had not realised the barriers that might be erected by the Israel customs people. I arranged to get a supply of lithium and identical-looking placebo capsules from Pfizer Drug Company, but these were held up at the customs for about a month until I paid an enormous duty on the placebo since it was not on their list of drugs that could be brought in without tax. I found a colleague at the Shaare Zedek Hospital who had an atomic absorption spectrophotometer, and was willing to do routine serum lithium determinations at cost. But he did not have the lamp needed for a cadmium standard. At this point I was exasperated with the Israel customs people, and had begun to understand that they would look the other way on humanitarian violations of their rules, so long as it did not appear on paper. So I had the appropriate materials purchased by the hospital and shipped to my mother who brought them in her handbag on her visit a few months after my arrival . . . Lithium treatment is now reasonably widespread in Israel, and the laboratory determination of serum lithium is no longer an exotic test, and I like to think that I helped this process along.[76]

Information about how lithium usage came to be established in the communist countries of eastern and central Europe is difficult to come by, but the situation in Czechoslovakia is probably not untypical. Shortly after the publication of Cade's original paper[77] on lithium, Dr L. Hanzlíček[78] and Dr Milos Vojtechovsky started to use lithium salts in Czechoslovakia, but the treatment was not continued because of the occurrence of toxic side effects. Dr Paul Grof, who joined the Psychiatric Research Institute in Prague in 1962, takes up the story:

The next move took place in 1965 when I went to visit Mogens Schou in Denmark and of course was very much turned on by him and his ideas. Perhaps I should mention a few events which led up to this. When I came to the Psychiatric Research Institute . . . the Psychopharmacology Department appeared spellbound by the double-blind in-patient studies. While they are very important, when they take over all research activities they become quite inflexible and, eventually, boring. Thus, to loosen the conceptual chains, and to put to use my interest in depression, I set up an out-patient follow-up clinic (Affective Disorders Clinic) independent of the in-patient predictable railroad. In psychopharmacological enthusiasm – and in hindsight a substantial naïvety – we set up a number of studies investigating the benefits of prophylactic treatments in recurrent affective disorders. That is, putative benefits, because we could not find any benefits, except perhaps for the psychological one for the therapist.

Thus, when Jules Angst brought to my attention the preliminary manuscript by Mogens Schou suggesting that the natural course of the illness can be profoundly changed by lithium salts I was absolutely skeptical. I felt quite sure that Schou must be wrong and would not have paid any attention to the report had it not been for Jules who knew Mogens well and felt that Mogens would not write about something he had not clearly observed himself. I decided to visit Mogens Schou and I believe I went to prove him wrong. However, the visit with Schou made me too curious to stop at that and I went back and started working systematically on the same group of patients that I had tried to treat prophylactically in vain for several previous years. I remember quite vividly the response my director had, when I told him upon my return about my decision to treat with lithium. He told me that I was dealing with a highly toxic substance and that if something were to go wrong I should not expect any help or support from him and should look for a job elsewhere.

On the other hand, I found great help from Dr Peter Zvolsky who was my colleague from medical school and who had worked at that time at Charles University Psychiatric Clinic. As there was no access to lithium serum levels, he managed to dig out an ancient flamephotometer, perhaps 20 years old, and started determining serum lithium levels. From my office the patients had to travel to him across the whole city, for nearly two hours, but they did not seem to mind once they realised that the treatment really worked. By 1967 we prepared our first reports in Czech and German and these were published in the subsequent year. It was within this context that in January 1967 Mogens Schou came to visit and gave a lecture at an annual psychopharmacological conference held at the small

Czechoslovak spa of Jesenik. After that he came to Prague and saw several of our patients with me in our office and consulted on difficult clinical problems.[79]

When Peter Zvolsky had been approached by Paul Grof about the problem of determining serum lithium levels he had readily agreed to help, but he soon found that there were formidable technical problems to be overcome.

> Never being a biochemist, I was at that time very provisionally in charge of our nearly non-existent biochemistry unit. Nevertheless, I thought that it was an interesting challenge. I went to the lab's cellar where I dug out an ancient flame photometer (Zeiss) which must have dated from the Second World War or early postwar times. I put it together, and after a short time we were able to determine levels of lithium ... with sufficient reliability, and the prophylactic treatment of manic–depressive patients in Czecho-slovakia had begun. ...
>
> The old apparatus from Zeiss worked quite satisfactorily for two or three years and then was replaced by a more adequate flame photometer from the same firm. It works well to this day. ...[80]

Paul Grof and Dr Karel Souček (who had been stimulated by the work and enthusiasm of Zvolsky) set up their own out-patient lithium clinics and commenced using lithium treatment systematically. At the present time, Czechoslovakia hosts a number of dedicated lithium research workers.[81]

In Roumania, the concept of the gouty diathesis was still flourishing in 1949; a product called Litinal, which contained lithium carbonate in an effervescent mixture to be made up with water and drunk at table, was widely available. It was withdrawn following the toxicity scare of 1949 and 1950, and the climate in Roumania became less conducive to the use of lithium salts in medical practice until the mid-1960s when Schou's work in Denmark became widely known. At this time, work commenced on the cellular metabolic aspects of lithium under G. Balan, Professor Marie Sibi and Dr L. Ababei at the Spitalul Clinic de Psihiatrie 'Socola' in Iaşi. Subsequently Dr G. Balan has become one of the best known lithium research workers in Roumania and lithium is now used in all the major medical centres in that country.

Future trends

Lithium salts are still comparatively inexpensive by comparison with other major psychoactive agents and for this reason are likely to be used to an increasing extent by the underdeveloped and developing countries of the Third World as their medical and psychiatric services become established and mental illness is more frequently diagnosed. Certainly, this is already happening in India, Egypt, the Philippines, certain central African countries, and in South America. In the People's Republic of China there has been a very recent expression of interest in developing lithium therapy services. Dr Yan Shanming, Head of the Department of Psychiatry at Zhenjiang Psychiatric Hospital, Jiangsu, has recently published a brief survey of lithium use in his country,[82] concluding that it is at present much underused. According to his estimate[83] the admission frequency for mania in a typical Chinese psychiatric hospital is about 10 per cent rather than the 1–3 per cent previously thought. If this becomes generally recognised there is likely to be a considerable increase in lithium use in China over the next few years. Hopefully, the results of this will become available outside China. As Yan Shanming notes:

We were so seclusive in the past 30 years that it was the first time in my life to have my report[84] on lithium published abroad.[85]

The further spread of lithium therapy will be facilitated by modern communication techniques, by the wider availability and greater variety of scientific journals, and by the continued efforts of those who, like Mogens Schou, have made it a major part of their work to publicise and explain the therapeutic benefits to be derived from this simple but powerful form of treatment.

9
Developments and crises

Lithium as an antidepressant

It is a well-known feature of the life history of any new medication that there should, over time, be a predictable shift in the way in which it is regarded. When therapeutic efficacy is first established, the tendency is to think of the medication as specific to the condition for which it is first used. Lithium was, right from the early days, regarded by many as a specific antimanic treatment. John Cade himself, in 1970, referred to 'my discovery of the specific antimanic effect of the lithium ion'.[1]

Later, however, the medication is tried for other conditions and if, for some of them, therapeutic benefit appears to be obtained, the claim for specificity of action comes under attack. Of course, it is possible that all the conditions susceptible to the effect of the new medication share some common underlying mechanism, and when this is realised or postulated the claims for therapeutic specificity are revived. More often, careful clinical trials reveal that the medication does not have clear-cut beneficial effects in as many conditions as was claimed, and this too lends support to the notion of specificity.

From a purely theoretical point of view, the issue of therapeutic specificity is an important one since it provides prima facie evidence of the aetiological or mechanistic distinctness (or otherwise) of disorders which, from their symptoms, might have been considered to have quite a different relationship. As far as lithium is concerned, its therapeutic efficacy against mania when used acutely, and its prophylactic properties against both mania and depression, raise the question of the link between these two aspects of affective dysfunction. The curious asymmetry between the acute and prophylactic actions of lithium as far as mania and depression were concerned did not go unremarked by those who were involved with lithium at an early stage in its history. After all, if lithium truly was effective both acutely and prophylactically against mania, but only prophylactically against depression, then this implied something very interesting, and potentially important, about the relationship between the two states. The first question which had to be asked, of course, was whether or not lithium really *was* ineffective when used acutely against any ongoing depressive state. First results seemed to indicate that this was indeed the case.

When Cade gave lithium to patients suffering from chronic depression[2] he found neither improvement nor impairment of their clinical condition, a conclusion also reached by others.[3] In fact, Noack and Trautner[4] actually suggested that lithium treatment might have made the depression rather worse.

In 1959, Schou gave a brief mention[5] to a study conducted but not published[6] on the therapeutic effects of lithium in endogenous depression. In a double-blind clinical trial on unipolar recurrent depressive patients, what was described as a 'rather clear-cut negative result' was obtained.[7]

Only in one out of twelve patients thus treated did the condition [depression] change synchronously with the medication: improvement during lithium periods and aggravation during placebo periods. But when lithium was administered to this patient during subsequent depressive phases, it was without any beneficial effect. The clinical changes observed in the eleven other patients could not with any probability be ascribed to lithium; administration of the drug resulted neither in improvement nor in aggravation of the depressions.[8]

Despite these negative findings, there were two early suggestions that lithium might, in certain cases, act as an acute antidepressant. Dr M. Vojtechovsky[9] in Czechoslovakia reported an improvement under lithium treatment in eight patients whose depression had proved unresponsive to electroconvulsive therapy, though a further six patients did not improve: this was in 1957. The following year, in Italy, a group led by Dr G. Andreani produced very similar findings,[10] with ten out of twenty-four severely depressed patients showing an apparently clear benefit from lithium treatment.

Since both these reports were published in languages other than English, they gained little currency outside their countries of origin. Even if they had been more generally available, however, it is doubtful they would have had much impact since, in terms of methodological soundness, they both left much to be desired. The question of spontaneous remission was, for example, left unanswered: this is a serious flaw in any work on a periodic illness such as depression.

It was around 1958 that a number of very effective antidepressant compounds were developed and marketed, and interest in the acute antidepressant properties of lithium understandably subsided, so that no reports of studies on the topic appeared in the literature until some ten years later when Ronald Fieve, in association with Stanley Platman and Robert

Plutchik[11] (all at the New York State Psychiatric Institute) reopened the issue, albeit in a very tentative fashion. In a study involving twenty-nine depressed patients a mild antidepressant action was accorded to lithium; the clinical trial was double-blind and methodologically sound in other ways, but still the conclusion was not without its qualification – the authors ended their report by suggesting that 'one cannot exclude the possibility that this mild antidepressant effect would be equally produced by any physiologically active substance'.[12] In other words, it might simply have been that the patients felt physiologically different and attributed this to being given an active agent: the belief that any agent with physiological effects must inevitably have therapeutic properties, may have been significant to convince the patients that improvement was taking place.

In a review of lithium therapy up to 1968, Schou concluded that the available observations indicated 'that in severe depression lithium is of little or no value'.[13]

The year 1968 was, however, a turning point, marked by a report[14] by Drs William Dyson and Myer Mendelson, both of the University of Pennsylvania Medical School, in which they gave detailed case histories of three patients treated successfully with lithium during a depressive episode, and noted similar success in two others. Whilst the study was an open, non-double-blind trial, and suffered from all the usual defects (e.g. the apparent lithium effect could simply have been the result of a spontaneous remission), the report nevertheless had an impact upon psychiatric opinion, not least because of the use of the term 'lithium responders'[15] to delineate a possible subgroup of depressive patients who might benefit from lithium treatment. Dyson, in association with Dr Joe Mendels, suggested[16] that the acute antidepressant effect of lithium might be restricted to bipolar, rather than unipolar, depressive states, a finding which lent further support to the notion of special lithium-responsive conditions. A year later, at the National Institute of Mental Health in Bethesda, Frederick Goodwin, Dennis Murphy and William Bunney added their voices[17] to the growing body of opinion that 'lithium has at least a partial antidepressant effect when used acutely in some patients'[18] but added that they did not advocate the general use of lithium as an antidepressant since 'extensive and controlled comparative studies are needed to determine if any subgroups of depressed patients respond more favourably to lithium than to conventional antidepressants'.[19]

Despite a number of negative reports,[20] the evidence for an acute antidepressant potential steadily grew. In 1972, Joe Mendels, working with Stephen Secunda and W. L. Dyson, showed in a double-blind crossover study,[21] that lithium and desipramine had equal effectiveness against depression in a small group of selected patients. Subsequent work by others[22] broadly supported this conclusion, and the situation rests more or less unchanged at the present time. As it was recently summarised:

It seems likely that lithium is a more useful treatment for acute depression than has previously been supposed, although this probably applies to bipolar rather than unipolar illness.[23]

Work on the possible acute antidepressant properties of lithium encountered the same kind of resistance that had attended other aspects of lithium research. Joe Mendels, who was on the receiving end of much of this opposition, has tried to analyse the reasons behind it.[24]

> It has long been my impression that the dominant hold of the biogenic amine hypothesis of affective disorders, with the view that there was an aminergic excess in mania and a deficiency in depression, led many of the leaders in this field to rigidly resist the notion that a single pharmacological treatment might be effective in both depression and mania. Given that lithium had been clearly established as effective in the treatment of acute mania, there was a considerable theoretical (and perhaps emotional) reluctance to seriously consider the possibility that it might have an antidepressant effect.
>
> I recall many discussions and arguments around this point in the late 1960s where we were beginning our work on the project. There was also considerable resistance to funding this type of research because many of the people who were involved in making decisions about grant support were heavily invested in the classic amine theory and appeared to me to resist the notions that we (and others) were beginning to advance. I remember the way in which our early claims and suggestions were casually dismissed. There was an absence of the usual scientific curiosity that surrounded many other new (and controversial) ideas at the time.[25]

Mendels and his group persevered, however:

> My colleagues and I allowed ourselves to prepare a number of discussions and reviews on this topic during the 1970s (although it is true that some of these were repetitive and therefore perhaps redundant) because of the relative paucity of new information and what I perceived as a need to 'hammer the point home' in the hope that it would be taken more seriously and subjected to more widespread and careful evaluation. . . .
>
> Now, the original concept of the biogenic amine hypothesis has been abandoned by almost everybody (except a few diehards) and has been replaced by more complex (and, at times, more ephemeral) concepts which may yet turn out to be compatible with the notion that the lithium ion is effective in both mania and depression. I must say that I have felt for some years that if we (my colleagues and I at Penn) had not argued these points on a rather repetitive basis the issues might not have achieved the degree of exposure that they did.[26]

Thanks largely to the efforts of people like Joe Mendels and his colleagues, there is now a firm body of information on the antidepressant potential of lithium. The early use of lithium as an acute antidepressant, in the context of its being a substance acting against conditions related to the uric acid diathesis,[27] particularly by Frederick Lange,[28] seems thus to have found at least partial vindication in the clinical findings of the post-Cade era.

Other uses for lithium

In addition to his investigations of manic patients, Cade had also included in his original study[29] a series of schizophrenic subjects. He found that some alleviation of their clinical symptoms occurred under lithium therapy, but suggested that this related more to the selective elimination of affective components of the illness than it did to fundamental schizophrenic mechanisms. Over the years there has been no appreciable change in this position and current thinking on the matter is that, as far as clinical benefits in schizophrenia are concerned, lithium is likely to be effective only in combined schizophrenic and affective dysfunctional states.[30]

It is curious just how many of the later developments of lithium therapy can be traced directly to the writings of John Cade. In his 1949 paper[31] Cade had commented that lithium treatment would be likely to be effective in the control of restless impulses and ungovernable tempers, conditions for which leucotomy had, at that time, been used with some success. It was not, however, until some twenty years later that reports began to appear confirming that, in both humans and animals, lithium did indeed seem to have a marked anti-aggressive action.

The early evidence of a possible anti-aggressive potential came in 1969 in the form of two brief case reports from Sweden.[32] Dr Anna-Lisa Annell and Drs Hans Forssman and Jan Wålinder indicated that in mentally defective patients showing aggressive or uncontrollable temper outbursts, improvement on lithium was quite remarkable. A year later, in Czechoslovakia, Drs T. Dostal and P. Zvolsky[33] found reduced aggressiveness and a lower incidence of undisciplined behaviour in severely mentally retarded adolescents treated with lithium, though the extent to which this was secondary to a more general improvement in underlying affective disturbances is difficult to say.

Thereafter, reports of successful lithium treatment of aggressive patients began to multiply. The first clinical trial of lithium in the control of aggression was conducted in 1971 by Professor Michael Sheard of Yale University School of Medicine,[34] using twelve prisoners in a maximum-security state prison in Somers, Connecticut. Sheard reported that aggressive affect ratings were significantly reduced during periods of lithium treatment, as also were incidences of over-physical and aggressive behaviour.

In the mid-1970s there were numerous similar reports, virtually all concluding that lithium was a useful anti-aggressive agent, but since that time there has been no sign to show that this is a major indication for the use of lithium, and it seems likely that clinicians prefer to rely upon environmental means of modifying, controlling or restraining aggression, rather than risk the possible consequences of lithium toxicity.

In 1974 there appeared three reports, all arising from a group of investigators under the general leadership of Dr Nathan Kline in the USA,[35] which promised a new and potentially quite exciting use for lithium salts. Kline and his associates had tried lithium as a possible treatment for alcoholism and first results were more than promising. The rationale behind the work was simple enough.

Many authors have stated that it is reasonable to assume that most alcoholics are suffering from depression. This statement raises the question as to whether or not control of the affective disturbance in these patients would influence their addiction.[36]

Lithium, as an established modifier of affect in the long term seemed an obvious candidate for the role of an alcoholism-alleviating or preventing agent, and so Kline and his colleagues set up a double-blind single crossover of seventy-three patients selected from the Alcoholic Treatment Program of the Veterans' Administration Hospital at Togus, Maine. The results were very encouraging. Not only were the patients' drinking habits changed in the right direction by lithium, but even amongst patients who had to be readmitted to hospital those receiving lithium treatment had fewer alcoholic episodes. Kline commented: 'We, frankly did not expect to find such a dramatic improvement following lithium treatment'.[37]

But how dramatic *was* the lithium effect? Out of the original seventy-three patients, only thirty completed the full experimental study, the remainder failing to comply with their medication instructions, and four out of the sixteen patients who continued their lithium treatment reported that they had had one or more episodes of disabling drinking. Nevertheless, the difference between the lithium and placebo groups was statistically significant and, moreover, the findings were in marked contrast to the only other report on the subject which had appeared five years earlier. Dr Hans Fries of Sweden, reviewing experience with lithium therapy gained over a three-year period in the Academic Hospital at Uppsala, noted[38] that only one patient out of seventeen treated with lithium for periodic alcoholism had shown any therapeutic benefit. He commented that 'most of the other patients in this group stopped taking the drug of their own accord when they did not experience an immediate effect'.[39]

The most interesting outcome of the work by Kline's group, however, did not lie so much in the clinical efficacy of lithium against alcoholism, as in the suggestion that when this occurred it did not seem to be related to a concomitant alleviation of depressive mood, as the original hypothesis had implied that it would. Kline played down this aspect of the findings:

Whether the improved behaviour of our patients was or was not related to depression is secondary. Primary is the fact that lithium may be a powerful ally in prevention of periodic or chronic drinking problems.[40]

Others, however, saw the possible dissociation of lithium effects on alcoholism and depression as potentially important from a theoretical point of view. In Finland, in 1973 Dr David Sinclair was working in the Research Laboratories of the State Alcohol Monopoly (Allco) in Helsinki. As part of his research on the factors affecting voluntary alcohol drinking in laboratory animals he had begun to examine the effects of various metals, starting with zinc. Because of its known effects on the central nervous system, lithium was amongst the first batch of metals that he chose to investigate, and a preliminary study showed that it strongly suppressed the alcohol intake of rats.[41] Then he became aware of the human studies.

A major factor encouraging me to further the research was the report by Nathan Kline and his co-workers that lithium was successful in the treatment of human alcoholics.[42]

At the same time that Sinclair was setting up his studies in Finland, Dr Andrew Ho was commencing similar work in the USA. Ho had been engaged in research on lithium and brain biogenic amines at the New York University Medical Center in collaboration with Dr Sam Gershon, and in 1972 his interest shifted to alcohol dependence, voluntary alcohol consumption, and alcohol withdrawal symptoms, in animals. He, like Sinclair, became aware of Kline's use of lithium in humans, and was encouraged to pursue his own investigations.[43]

Since the early reports of 1974, however, very little follow-up work has been done on lithium in alcoholism. In 1977 Dr Alec Coppen and a small group of British investigators based at West Park Hospital, Epsom, published the results of their own study which confirmed the general conclusion reached by Kline:

It is clear that there are a considerable number of alcoholic patients who would show a substantial advantage in long-term lithium therapy.[44]

Why, then, did lithium treatment for alcoholism never become widely established? In the first place, the drop-out rate from treatment was always high (usually greater than 50 per cent), making it an unreliable form of medication. Secondly, doubts were expressed about toxic complications. Andrew Ho says that he became worried about the potential hazards of indiscriminate use of lithium in alcoholism, 'especially since little is known about its interaction toxicities'.[45] It was just this issue that gave pause to David Sinclair.

The initial studies had seemed to suggest that lithium had a simple, uniform influence in suppressing alcohol drinking, and previous research in other fields had shown that with the proper control it could be used safely. As a simple and safe substance, it could be used as a tool in the study of alcohol drinking and as a treatment for human alcohol abuse even in the absence of an understanding of how it works. Unfortunately, additional investigations showed that it was neither simple nor always safe. Several circumstances were discovered in which lithium inexplicably did not reduce the alcohol consumption of rats or even increased it. Furthermore, lithium interacted with alcohol intoxication, and its own toxicity, at least in rats, increased as a function of the animals' previous ethanol experience. Although these questions regarding the complexity of lithium's actions on ethanol drinking and its toxicity could be seen as proper subjects for future research, and indeed must be resolved if lithium is to be widely used with human alcoholics, their resolution is, I feel, dependent upon a proper understanding of the mechanisms regulating alcohol drinking and intoxication. Consequently, I have returned to more basic alcohol research and dropped the study of lithium until there is a better foundation for understanding its interactions with ethanol.[46]

Certainly there was not a great deal of enthusiasm generated amongst grant-awarding bodies for the support of work on alcoholism and lithium. Sinclair had a grant proposal rejected by an American award committee. 'There were', he says, 'probably many reasons for the rejection, but one explanation I heard was that lithium – alcohol research had been over-popularised.'[47] Nevertheless, Sinclair added that he had no evidence that this did create a resistance among the members of the granting committee and he is inclined to believe that it was not an important factor in the decision.

With the exception of one or two relatively rare conditions (such as, for example, cluster headache[48]) the only unequivocal indication for the use of lithium in psychiatry remains in recurrent affective disorder – acutely for mania and prophylactically for mania and depression. All other developments have failed, for one reason or another, to progress beyond a certain point and remain subject to discussion and dispute.

Technical developments

All the developments in the conduct of lithium therapy, which have taken place at a technical level, have been directed towards the maintenance of serum lithium concentrations within safe and effective limits. To this end there have been advances in the way in which lithium compounds are administered, and in the monitoring of serum levels once administration has occurred. The formulation of sustained-release lithium products has been an important development, though there remains much debate on the relative efficacies of such substances and the available ordinary, non-sustained-release products.[49]

The necessity for careful serum lithium monitoring has been an issue which has concerned Dr Amdi Amdisen of Aarhus University Psychiatric Hospital, Denmark, for the greater part of his professional career, and it is with his name that the generally followed guidelines are associated. Amdisen had been a medical student at the Medical Biochemical Institute of Aarhus University and in 1959, preparatory to entering general practice, was completing his psychiatric training when the physician in charge asked him to take special care of the treatment of a manic–depressive man.

> This patient had shown an unquestionably good response to lithium treatment but now was in a peculiar state not seen before at this psychiatric clinic. I soon got the suspicion that he was lithium-intoxicated and from Mogens Schou, whom I knew from the time I had spent at the Biochemistry Institute, I got a copy of Cade's paper from 1949, and my suspicion was then proved to be correct.[50]

Amdisen joined Mogens Schou's unit and trained to become a clinical chemist.

> From the very beginning my interest was to make the lithium treatment more safe and more efficient, primarily through mapping out the serum kinetics of lithium and trying to find an efficient monitoring system.
>
> The biochemical and basic biological properties of the lithium ion have never been in the centre of my interest. From the start I regarded lithium as used in psychiatry as a toxic drug with a huge variety of toxic effects within the living cells and cell system, and I have never believed that such a general toxicity could give a clue to the biochemical mechanisms behind the manic–depressive diseases.
>
> However, from the beginning it was clear to me that the lithium therapy was of critical importance to patients in whom it works, and also from the beginning I have been aware of its risks. My interest has, in short, been to try to make a safety net beneath the lithium treatment.[51]

The empirical and technical background to serum monitoring was already available in the pioneering work of Trautner,[52] but Amdisen developed the procedures further, drawing attention particularly to the rather unpredictable time-course of serum concentrations of lithium within the first few hours of ingesting a lithium tablet, and also emphasising the need for serum levels to be monitored at a fixed and rigorously standardised time interval after ingestion of the last tablet. He developed the idea of the twelve-hour standard serum lithium level (12h-stSLi) as an attempt to formalise this aspect of monitoring dose levels.

With the advent of atomic absorption spectroscopy, and the ready availability of both atomic absorption and flame emission spectrophotometric equipment in hospitals, the clinical use of serum lithium measurement rapidly became established as a mainstay of responsible patient management.[53] In a way, this technical development has probably had paradoxical effects upon the spread and acceptance of lithium therapy. To the extent that it made the treatment safer, by allowing the early detection of potentially dangerous rises in serum levels of lithium, by giving rise to established guidelines for dosage control, and by encouraging a closer understanding of lithium kinetics within the clinical therapeutic context, serum monitoring made lithium therapy acceptable to clinicians who would not otherwise have taken the risk of using a known toxic substance. On the other hand, the necessity for carrying out serum determinations – particularly in the early stages of treatment, but also at regular intervals thereafter – has certainly discouraged the introduction of this treatment in countries where there is no ready access to appropriate equipment. Even in the developed nations, lithium therapy is properly regarded as a treatment for which hospital supervision is required during the period of its establishment, and for that reason there may well be reluctance amongst medical practitioners not based in a hospital, to consider lithium treatment as a viable, or at least an attractive, option. Attempts to devise simpler procedures for dosage monitoring in order to facilitate the introduction of lithium therapy in areas where frequent sampling of blood is not an easy matter, have not generally proved satisfactory. Urine lithium levels are not sufficiently stable to be used for this purpose,[54] though saliva levels show rather more promise.[55]

Crises

There have been several times in the history of lithium therapy when it appeared that the treatment might be associated with problems of a magnitude sufficient to threaten seriously its viability as a generally available, long-term solution to the problem of recurrent mood disorders. Each of these crises led to a ripple of unease amongst those engaged in administering lithium treatment, and each has left a scar on the reputation of lithium therapy, but the therapy has survived more or less intact. It is not possible to go into the history of these crises in any great detail but the more salient features may be quickly summarised.

Like the crisis caused by the toxicity panic of the late 1940s and early 1950s,[56] the subsequent difficulties experienced by lithium therapy have all related to matters of intoxication or side effects. In 1969 Dr Göran Sedvall and his colleagues at St Göran's Hospital, Stockholm, wrote an interesting article in which they raised the issue of long-term side effects in lithium therapy.

Lithium has been used successfully in the treatment of manic–depressive disease for almost twenty years. Some patients have received the drug daily for more than ten years. Considering what is known about the chronic toxicity of other drugs, it is remarkable that practically no reports of any chronic side effects of lithium salts in psychiatric patients have been communicated. Neither does there seem to have been any systematic study of the chronic toxicity of lithium in experimental animals in the doses used in the clinic. For these reasons it is very important to be constantly on the look-out for the appearance of unusual effects during lithium therapy.[57]

The particular unusual effect noted by Sedvall and his group was related to the functioning of the thyroid. For a number of years psychiatrists in Scandinavia had been aware that there might be a thyroid problem in some patients receiving lithium. For example, Dr Amdi Amdisen had chanced upon some evidence to this effect in 1967.

One of my friends, a surgeon, had been working with transfer of penicillin from the mother to the foetus, and I tried to get an impression of lithium. My very first newborn child from a lithium-treated mother had a very high serum lithium concentration and, furthermore, a huge struma, which almost strangled the little girl. This gave rise to my interest in lithium-produced goitre.[58]

Mogens Schou, moreover, had suggested in 1968 that lithium might be involved in thyroid enlargement; but he did not commit himself firmly on the matter.[59] Sedvall's group, however, produced clear evidence. In 1968 they started a study to investigate lithium effects on the thyroid gland, their interest being prompted by an almost accidental finding that in some of their lithium-treated patients there was an unusually low level of serum protein-bound iodine. Their results, published in 1969, confirmed that this effect was reproducible, and also showed that it reversed upon withdrawal of lithium.

The work of the Stockholm group prompted others to look into the matter. Amdisen published his observations on the development of goitre in the newborn child (and also in the mother).[60] It is, in fact, difficult to assign precise priorities in this matter, since the Swedish study was not published until 1969 whereas Amdisen's findings had appeared a year earlier.[61] Sedvall and his co-workers had, however, also given details of their work on serum protein-bound iodine in 1968,[62] and so it seems that this is an example of simultaneous but independent discovery by two distinct groups of investigators.

After these early reports, the occurrence of thyroid disturbance – usually goitre or hypothyroidism, but occasionally hyperthyroidism – became a matter of quite common observation in the literature.[63] Since the first studies had shown the thyroid effects to be generally benign, and since subsequent work demonstrated that the effects could be easily controlled by thyroxine administration (when reducing the lithium dose either does not work or is not advisable), what might have been an awkward situation for lithium therapy proved in the event to be no more than a minor irritation.

What was potentially a rather more serious problem arose in 1969. In that year, Dr Morton Weinstein and Dr Michael Goldfield, both of the Langley Porter Neuropsychiatric Institute in San Francisco, published an account[64] of a woman who had been given lithium treatment throughout pregnancy, and who subsequently gave birth to an entirely normal baby son. In their account, Weinstein and Goldfield described graphically their anxieties when they discovered that the patient (referred to as B.L.) was eight to twelve weeks pregnant and still taking lithium.

In the month that followed this disclosure she suffered from morning sickness and her effective lithium intake was often in doubt. The prospect of a therapeutic abortion was discussed with her and her new husband, but both declined to consider it. Despite the turmoil and uncertainty intro-duced into her life by the pregnancy and her precipitate marriage, her mood remained neutral and her behaviour became more appropriate; she began a new job as soon as the subsidence of her morning sickness permitted.

We and B.L. were then faced with the choice, on the one hand, of continuing her seemingly effective lithium programme past the first trimester of her pregnancy and take an unknown risk with the fetus, or terminating B.L.'s lithium and taking a grave risk with her emotional state on the eve of delivery and motherhood. Further, we could not evaluate the possibility that the teratogenicity of lithium for the human fetus, *if any*, might *already* have had its effect. Our urgent review of the English-language literature concerning the teratogenicity of lithium in humans produced no data of value except for Schou's brief but reassuring comment,[65] and a telephone discussion with the appropriate officials of the Food and Drug Administration failed to lead us to clear evidence of teratogenicity in mammals. We conferred at length and in detail with B.L., her husband, and her parents, giving them as much information as we ourselves had concerning the risks and advantages of continuing lithium treatment. Our decision was to recommend its continuation. B.L. and her family agreed.[66]

As a result of this experience, Weinstein and Goldfield set up what they referred to as the American Register of Lithium Babies to be maintained at the Langley Porter Institute. They requested that reports of pregnancies under lithium treatment should be communicated to them for inclusion in the Register. In Denmark, Mogens Schou was already collecting details of pregnancies and births which had occurred under lithium therapy, and had set up the Scandinavian Register of Lithium Babies; he was immediately contacted by Weinstein and Goldfield. Schou suggested that the Scandinavian Register should be combined with the American Register. Dr André Villeneuve, of Quebec, who had started a Canadian Register of Lithium Babies after the establishment of the American Register, also put his material into the common pool. There thus arose what came to be called the International Register of Lithium Babies,[67] maintained primarily by Morton Weinstein until his tragic and untimely death in 1979.[68] At the time of Weinstein's last report[69] the International Register contained 225 cases, of which twenty-five concerned congenitally malformed infants. By far the greatest number of malformations related to the cardiovascular system, with Ebstein's anomaly being 150 times more frequent than in the general population.

Of course, as Schou has consistently contended,[70] there was probably always a tendency for the Register to receive reports of more malformed than normal babies, but nevertheless the finding of an association between lithium treatment and foetal abnormalities was too clear to be ignored and could well have had a detrimental effect upon the acceptance of lithium therapy. This was a particularly strong possibility since the affective dysfunctions for which lithium is used tend to occur most frequently during the procreative years. That there was, in fact, relatively little impact upon the development of lithium therapy is almost certainly due to the provision by Morton Weinstein and Michael Goldfield of a set of sensible guidelines for rational lithium treatment when pregnancy either occurs or is considered a possibility.[71]

Probably the most serious challenge of all to the continued use of long-term lithium therapy was posed by the suggestion that continued treatment might be associated with an increased risk of renal damage. It had been known for a long time, mainly from work with animals, that lithium toxicity could manifest itself in functional, and sometimes structural, changes in the kidney,[72] and in the late 1960s these became the subject of considerable clinical interest, particularly at the hands of Dr Amdi Amdisen.

> About 1967 my youngest child had grown up to seven years of age and my wife resumed her work as a nurse. It happened to be work within our local haemodialysis centre. Through this I got a certain knowledge of haemodialysis. Simultaneously, my name became known among colleagues in our region of the country so that very often they contacted me directly if they had any problems with their lithium-treated patients. In this way, I became acquainted with all degrees of lithium intoxication and it was natural for me to try to treat a case of severe lithium intoxication with haemodialysis and during this treatment to follow the lithium concentration within the spinal fluid. . . .
>
> As a result of a still increasing frequency of lithium-intoxicated patients, I got into close cooperation with my wife's chief at the Nephrology

Unit and this gave rise to the recognition of the practical importance of the discrimination between acute renal toxicity and chronic renal toxicity of lithium as it was currently used within psychiatry.[73]

Over the next few years what has been referred to as 'the kidney scare'[74] developed rapidly. In 1977 two reports appeared which brought matters to a head:[75] in these, Dr H. E. Hansen, together with Dr Amdisen, Dr J. Hestbech and other colleagues, drew attention to chronic functional and morphological changes which occurred in the kidney of patients after extended treatment with lithium. In particular, disturbances in renal concentrating ability and glomerular sclerosis were found to be far more common in the lithium-treated patients than in age-matched controls, and there was a doubling of interstitial connective tissue. Other reports of kidney damage followed, and inevitably the question of the safety of lithium therapy had eventually to be posed:

Are we buying the mental health of lithium-treated manic–depressive patients at the expense of their kidney function and survival? Should we perhaps stop using lithium? Should we avoid using it for periods longer than a few years?[76]

The confidence of psychiatrists in lithium treatment was badly shaken.

The reports made a profound impression on the psychiatric world. There was a drastic fall in the number of patients started on lithium and many patients were taken off lithium treatment on which they had done well. This resulted in relapses, and suicides are known to have occurred.[77]

As more information was assembled, both from patients and from studies using animal subjects, the whole issue of lithium-induced renal damage became increasingly complicated. For one thing, some investigators could find very little functional evidence of renal changes,[78] and there was a report from a group of investigators at the Royal Melbourne Hospital, Australia,[79] to the effect that renal structural lesions similar to those found in lithium-treated patients (but without impairment of tubular concentrating ability) could also be detected in patients suffering from recurrent affective disorders and treated with psychotropic drugs but not yet with lithium – thus raising the possibility that the lesions were either produced by other agents or were typically associated with affective dysfunction.

The crisis over renal damage was never resolved in a completely satisfactory manner: it simply faded as a matter of major concern since, as Professor F. A. Jenner remarked, 'it seems to be agreed by nephrologists ... that widespread lithium treatment does not lead to large numbers of people presenting with chronic renal failure requiring transplants.'[80] While no one really denied, or does deny, that some degree of nephropathy is associated with lithium treatment, the degree to which it occurs is quite evidently less than is produced by certain other substances, such as the heavy metals, and on most assessments would appear to be tolerable given the benefits conferred by lithium in other directions. Schou and Vestergaard have given the frankest appraisal of the current position:

> The observation that lithium may produce, or accentuate, nonspecific morphologic changes in the kidneys and that lithium treatment may lead to impairment of renal water reabsorption, not always fully reversible, does not seem to justify radical changes in the use of lithium on proper psychiatric indications. . . . Additional kidney function tests such as serial determinations of serum creatinine, determination of glomerular filtration rate, measurement of urine volume, and determination of concentrating ability may be carried out as extra safety measures and for research purposes in suitably equipped hospitals, but they can hardly be considered mandatory.[81]

This view is one endorsed in general terms by H. E. Hansen:

> It is unlikely that lithium-induced nephropathy will cause severe renal failure or terminal uraemia. The changes in renal function which may develop during long-term lithium treatment should not result in unnecessary anxiety and do not contra-indicate lithium treatment.[82]

Amdisen, whilst feeling that the whole issue may have been blown up out of all proportion, cautions against an over-reaction leading to a dismissal of what he sees as a very real problem:

> The 'kidney scare' was a panic reaction *among psychiatrists* which was unreasonably hysterical and undoubtedly caused by insufficient knowledge about the pathology of the kidneys: an exaggerated acute reaction which currently is on its way to the opposite unreasonable reaction, namely a pooh-pooh of the lithium-produced kidney impairments – the latter again because of missing competence concerning nephrology.[83]

He makes the further point that:

> Most psychiatrists interested in lithium have not fully recognised that it is not the polyuria or the concentrating ability alone, or the histopathological changes in the kidneys alone, which raise the consideration, but the combination of reduced renal concentrating ability and the interstitial nephropathy.
>
> Our opinion is still the same as it was in 1976–1977. The chronic renal toxicity of lithium as it is currently used requires certain, rather limited, extra control procedures. But there was no reason and there is no reason, for either panic or hysteria.[84]

As with virtually all new medications, many problems have been encountered in the use of lithium. Only a few have been sufficiently serious to pose a potential threat to the viability of lithium therapy; others have appeared at first dramatic, only to be rapidly resolved. An alarmingly high incidence of sudden deaths amongst lithium patients at the Affective Disorders Clinic of the New York University Medical Center, reported in 1978 by Dr Baron Shopsin,[85] might well have led to many patients being taken off lithium had it not been for the fact that his research team of geneticists found that all the patients who died had at least one first-degree male relative within the same age range who had also died as a result of cardiac dysfunction, albeit not suddenly. Lithium, it appeared, might accentuate or uncover an underlying cardiac deficiency. By recognising this possibility, and by carefully screening all patients for familial predisposition to cardiac insufficiency, this potential of lithium for harm can be eliminated as a major problem in therapy.

Looking back over the fortunes of lithium therapy in the thirty or so years that it has been used on any scale, it is remarkable how few major developments or crises have occurred. One might have expected that a drug with such an apparently powerful therapeutic effect on a major psychiatric disorder, would find uses in a wide variety of other conditions – certainly on the basis of experience with other agents such as chlorpromazine and haloperidol. This has not happened, and lithium remains a medication having relatively specific clinical indications. Such developments as have occurred have been mainly in the direction of better patient management and the avoidance of toxicity or side effects. It would not have been unreasonable to have expected more crises, too. The toxicity panic of the first few years of lithium therapy's existence,[86] seemed to presage a much more stormy passage than was, in the event, experienced. The crises, when they occurred, were hardly serious enough to warrant the use of the term. There were, of course, episodes other than those which have been referred to in this chapter, which seemed to call into question the safety of lithium treatment given under certain circumstances, but all were minor and were readily resolved by adjustment to the dosage regime or by appropriate prior screening of patients; a few were traceable to errors of medical judgement on the part of the supervising clinician.

It seems fair to conclude that the progress of lithium therapy has been smoother, from a purely clinical point of view, than one might have anticipated; it is, therefore, all the more curious that, of all available psychiatric drug treatments lithium therapy is still the one treated with most suspicion and mistrust by so many clinicians, and even with outright and overt hostility by a few. The legacy of the toxicity panic and the therapeutic myth allegation are both evident and resilient.

10
The future

If the task of disentangling the historical threads in the lithium story is difficult, that of predicting what the future may hold for lithium therapy is almost impossible. It is, in any case, an exercise to be undertaken with circumspection: only the most incautious individual would suppose there to be any certainties in medical research. The probabilities, however, are there for all to see.

The therapeutic profile

The title which lithium holds to being the treatment of first choice for recurrent affective disorders seems to be secure; and whilst in the acute treatment of mania and in the prophylactic treatment of both unipolar and bipolar affective illness there may eventually be some greater precision in specifying the parameters which govern effective treatment, it seems likely that lithium therapy will consolidate its position in the psychiatrist's armamentarium.

The situation with the acute treatment of depressive illness is rather less clear. It certainly seems as though there is a subgroup of depressed patients who are responders to lithium, but unless they are also refractory to other forms of antidepressant medication it is improbable that lithium will ever be generally considered as the first-choice treatment for such patients. Nevertheless, clarification of what distinguishes a responder from a non-responder in this respect could provide useful information about both the nature of depressive illness and the criteria upon which the clinical decision to use lithium should be based.

At the present time, there seems to be little future for lithium as a medication in the control of schizophrenia, except when there is an accompanying affective component of a fairly distinct nature.

There are several conditions for which lithium has already been used – often with mixed success – and for which some degree of future use seems possible. In general, any condition characterised by a periodic course seems to be a potential candidate for lithium therapy, and amongst these periodic cluster headache will continue to be treated with lithium. The simple analogy of a non-affective periodic syndrome with the periodicity of recurrent affective disorders is not an infallible guide to therapeutic success, however; the results of lithium trials in premenstrual tension, for example, have been disappointing.

All-in-all the therapeutic profile of lithium in psychiatry seems likely to remain much as it appears at the present time.

Factors in therapeutic outcome

If one were to point to a single area of lithium research in which the findings hold particular promise, not only for the development of lithium therapy itself but for our wider understanding of psychiatric disorder, it would probably be to work on the problem of predicting which patients will be lithium responders and which non-responders. In recent years, increasing attention has been given to the question of 'biological markers', or indicators (physiological, biochemical, psychological), that characterise certain individuals as being more (or less) likely than others either to suffer from, or to be cured of, particular psychiatric conditions.

Within lithium research a number of such markers have been tentatively proposed, though none has proven to be a perfect predictor of lithium responsiveness. However, developments are proceeding so rapidly in this field that it seems well within the bounds of possibility that one or more fairly specific predictors of therapeutic outcome will be established in the next few years. The impact which this would have upon the rational treatment of patients can well be imagined.

A related issue concerns patient compliance with medication. This, of course, is only one aspect of the more general topic of patient–physician relationships, but it is particularly important since it is non-compliance with the treatment regime which probably accounts for the greater number of the reported incidences of lithium non-response. It may well be that by paying greater attention to the social and psychological support which is given to the patient who is starting lithium treatment, the number dropping out of treatment may be greatly reduced. This, in its turn, would undoubtedly enhance the image of lithium therapy in the eyes of clinicians, though one has to bear in mind that the economics of providing adjunctive support of this kind may prove to be unrealistic.

The therapeutic routine

As specialised affective disorders clinics become established, the routine of lithium therapy will inevitably come under closer scrutiny. This could have two quite opposite effects. On the one hand, the concentration of research facilities and personnel within a single clinical unit could encourage the use of a broad range of screening test procedures, primarily on a research basis, to identify factors associated with therapeutic effectiveness or lithium toxicity; on the other hand, as knowledge accumulates on which of these factors are important, there will be a tendency for some tests to be dropped and others to be given greater priority. In the short-term, then, an increase in adjunctive testing may occur, but this, if it does take place, will be the prelude to the development of a more rational, and less extensive, test battery.

Serum lithium monitoring techniques are already rapid and accurate and any technical advances in this direction are unlikely to affect clinical practice to any appreciable extent. There may, however, be changes in attitudes towards serum level testing in general: there are those who feel that regular serum monitoring could be de-emphasised and that incipient toxicity could be determined on the basis of prodromal signs; others, however, concerned about possible long-term kidney damage, are of the opinion that the trend should be towards prescribing maintenance doses giving lower serum levels than has tended in the past to be the case, and for this to be done effectively it is necessary not only to have frequent serum monitoring, but for such measurements to be done in a rigorously standardised manner. Which of these approaches will gain ascendancy depends partly upon what kinds of resources are made available, but mainly upon new information linking serum lithium levels to the occurrence of long-term side effects.

There is a constant search for newer and more effective formulations, based mainly upon the assumption that the best results – and certainly the ones associated with fewest side effects – are to be obtained when serum lithium levels are maintained at as stable a level as possible. This may not, of course, be an entirely warranted assumption, but as long as it remains the current view, there will be a preference for lithium formulations which have sustained-release properties, and one may expect to see some developments along these lines, utilising some of the newer pharmaceutical techniques for the slow release of drugs.

Toxicity and side effects

Where side effects and toxic reactions are concerned, it is inevitable that interest will be sustained over the next few years. Renal effects will be followed with great interest, of course, and it is possible that a set of guidelines will be developed which will ensure that the risk of long-term renal damage is minimised.

The endocrine side effects of lithium, particularly in relation to thyroid gland activity, are by now so well established that there will probably not be a great deal new in this area, except perhaps for an elucidation of the underlying physiological processes.

The control of lithium-induced tremor is a perennial problem and there may be some progress here. Other classes of side effect tend to be relatively rare or transient and one may suppose that their management will continue to be mainly by dosage reduction or by the complete withdrawal of lithium.

The treatment of children, adolescents and the elderly always poses special problems where drugs are concerned. There are good reasons for avoiding drug therapy in children if at all possible, and this is particularly true of any drug treatment which is likely to have to be continued over an extended period; in general, lithium has not been widely used in the younger age range. However, as confidence grows in lithium amongst clinicians, it may well happen that lithium comes to be seen as a useful adjunct to the management of aggressive children, particularly when concomitant mental retardation leads to difficulties in establishing new behaviour patterns using standard training methods.

Psychological approaches

Recent years have seen a tendency for psychological investigations of lithium to be accorded a more prominent place in discussions of the theoretical bases of lithium treatment, and this is a trend which will undoubtedly continue and could lead to exciting future developments.

One of the most curious aspects of the lithium story from the point of view of the psychopharmacologist concerns the role which animal behaviour studies have played (or rather have failed to play) in the development of the practice and rationale of therapy. This stands in marked contrast to the situation with such agents as chlorpromazine and the various clinically useful benzodiazepines which have been subjected to a veritable investigative onslaught by psychologists and others using behavioural test situations and animal subjects.

There are several reasons why lithium should have been relatively neglected in this respect. In the first place, being an agent introduced into therapy at a time when drug control regulations were much less stringent than is now the case, lithium was not exposed to the battery of behavioural tests which are now required to determine likely effectiveness, before it was administered to patients and its actual effectiveness directly established: once that was accomplished, there may have seemed little point in expending time and energy in performing confirmatory laboratory studies.

Secondly, the toxicity panic led to effective removal of lithium from the psychopharmacological scene at a time when the behavioural analysis of drug action was experiencing something of a boom – in the early and mid-1950s; instead, attention was focused on chlorpromazine, the amphetamines, reserpine, and some of the newer anti-anxiety and antidepressant agents. By the time that lithium became generally acceptable again, the interest in behavioural work had undergone a subtle, but important, shift from fundamental investigation of mechanisms of action to the design of batteries of screening tests aimed at discovering new drugs to fulfil the burgeoning demand on the world pharmaceutical market. The majority of such screening tests were validated against existing drugs of known and established therapeutic efficacy and had, therefore, an inbuilt bias to discover agents with the same, or similar, modes of action. When lithium was subjected to these screening tests it tended to give negative results,[1] leading to the view that it was behaviourally inert when a more thoughtful interpretation might have been that its mode of action was probably different (either qualitatively or quantitatively) from those of the drugs used in setting up the screening tests in the first place. The inactive nature of lithium received further support from studies showing that, unlike chlorpromazine for example, it had little effect on the conscious experience of normal human volunteers.[2]

All this bolstered the notion that lithium was a specific medication for affective dysfunction, operating to correct or to offset some presumed illness-specific lesion. Since the lesion was, by definition, absent in animals and normal volunteers, the absence of behavioural effects of lithium outside the clinical context was both expected and explicable.

Nevertheless, it remained an awkward fact that John Cade's reintroduction of lithium into medical practice[3] had itself been based upon an observed effect on the behaviour of guinea-pigs, and by the early 1970s a few suggestions began to appear in the literature to the effect that lithium did seem to have some impairing action on activity levels – but the observations tended to be derived from experimental studies planned for other purposes, and the evidence was thus patchy and inconclusive.

The first clear report of an effect of lithium on the activity of animals appeared in February 1972.[4] Writing in *Nature*, Dr Neil Johnson and a colleague, Miss Serena Wormington, argued that despite the generally negative findings up to that time 'it would, nevertheless, be surprising if a drug of such apparent therapeutic efficacy had no effect on animals' and they therefore used a test apparatus which had previously been shown to be highly sensitive to low concentrations of psychoactive drugs. They succeeded in demonstrating that lithium seemed to affect the response of rats to external stimulation, and Johnson subsequently confirmed this finding in later studies.[5] The hypothesis was put forward[6] that lithium impaired the central analysis of around threshold levels of sensory input; from this a model of manic–depression was derived, based upon a dysfunction of information analysis.[7]

One might have thought that this would have aroused some comment, but in fact the work passed virtually unnoticed. There is, for reasons which are in part understandable, some reluctance on the part of psychiatrists to accord much weight to theoretical propositions based on work with animals; the information is felt to be of only indirect relevance to humans.

More recently, however, work on human subjects[8] has led to views being expressed about lithium which accord almost precisely with those put forward on the basis of animal work several years previously, and at the International Lithium Conference held in New York in June 1978, Johnson commented:[9]

> It is gratifying, now that human studies are at last being carried out, that the clear implications of the early animal studies are receiving strong support, and it encourages one to believe that animal studies will continue to have utility within the general area of lithium research.[10]

That remains the hope; the concurrence of the results of studies on animals and on humans, places statements about lithium action within a general biological context and at a level transcending species differences. Moreover, the establishment of psychological models of the way in which lithium produces its therapeutic effects has a clear value to psychiatrists who may find the notions so expressed more immediately understandable and relevant to their clinical activities than those used to propound biochemical or physiological models.

There is already a sound body of experimental studies on animal behaviour and lithium, and the opportunity now lies open for this encouraging beginning to be developed and capitalised upon.

Epilogue

The basic groundwork for future work on lithium has been firmly laid and we may expect that the opportunity will be taken to discover more about this curious element. It seems unlikely that dramatic new developments will take place; the process is more likely to be one of assimilating what is already known about lithium into the general body of models of affective disorders, and of seeking further specific information to test and to choose between the various alternative theoretical positions.

In short, the future for lithium seems to be more of (more or less) the same, but with maybe a shift of emphasis here and there. On the whole, and despite its ups and downs, the lithium story has been one of success, and in the coming years we shall no doubt see lithium therapy being less and less discussed in a critical manner as it establishes itself as a tried and trusted remedy alongside others.

Lithium has come a long way since the day in 1818 when a Brazilian nobleman stooped to pick up some strange pieces of rock lying on a tiny windswept island off the coast of Sweden, and placed them carefully amongst his other specimens. The historical progression from that moment to the establishment of lithium salts as powerful agents in the fight against mental illness has been a torturous and at times unexpected one. It may, perhaps, be seen as ironic that lithium should owe its central place in modern psychiatric medicine to a series of chance discoveries and, in the early years at least, erroneous hypotheses, but to conclude from this that the whole thing was just an enormous piece of luck does less than justice to the enquiring spirit, scientific integrity, and perspicacity of the relatively small band of investigators who, each in their own way, took the story one step further. They may have made mistakes, reached the wrong conclusions, misinterpreted or gone beyond their data, but it was all done in good faith and only with the omiscience of hindsight can we find fault: at the time their ideas were the springs from which new concepts and new theories flowed. Above all they kept lithium in the mainstream of medical practice so that when the time was ripe and the world was ready, the true nature of lithium could be revealed and understood.

Notes and references

1 The discovery of lithium

1. Joze Bonifacio de Andrada e Silva was born in Brazil on 13 June 1763, and received his higher education at the University of Coimbra in Portugal where he subsequently took up a post teaching metallurgy. He returned to Brazil in 1819 to take an active part in political life there, playing a leading role in establishing the country's constitution, but was subsequently exiled for a time and lived in France. On the abdication of Emperor Dom Pedro I, de Andrada went back to Brazil once more and became guardian to the heirs to the Brazilian throne. He died in Brazil, near Rio de Janeiro, on 6 April 1838.
2. De Andrada, J. B. (1800) 'Kurze Angabe der Eigenschaften und Kennzeichen einiger neuen Fossilien aus Schweden und Norwegen, nebst einingen chemischen Bemerkungen über dieselben', *Scherer's Allgemeine Journal der Chemie*, **4**, 28–39.
3. There is frequently much confusion concerning the spelling of Swedish names in reports published in the early 1800s. 'Svedenstjerna', for example, was spelt 'Swedenstierna' by E. D. Clarke (see note 4) and 'Sudenstierna' by N.-L. Vauquelin (see note 9).
4. Edward Daniel Clarke (1769–1822) was a renowned traveller and wrote extensively about his journeys to many parts of the world. A founder member of the Cambridge Philosophical Society, and Professor of Mineralogy in the University of Cambridge, he published reports on many different mineral types.
5. Clarke, E. D. (1818) 'Account of some remarkable minerals recently brought to this country from the island of Jean Maven in the Greenland seas, north latitude 71°. Also a description and analysis of a substance called petalite from Sweden', *Annals of Philosophy*, **11**, 194–98.
6. Spelt 'Dandrada' by Clarke.
7. Clarke, 'Account of some remarkable minerals', 198 (note 5).
8. Nicholas-Louis Vauquelin (1763–1829) was a man of humble origins who rose from being an apothecary's apprentice in Rouen, to become a member of the Legion d'Honneur, Director of the Ecole Spéciale de Pharmacie, Director of the Jardin des Plantes, and Professor in the Paris Medical Faculty.
9. Vauquelin, N.-L. (1817) 'Note sur une nouvelle espèce d'alcali minéral', *Annales de Chimie et de Physique*, **2**, 284–88.
10. Ibid., 284.
11. Johan August Arfwedson (1792–1841) was a Swede born into a prosperous family. He trained in the principles of mining, and at the age of 25, whilst serving in the Royal Bureau of Mines at Stockholm, undertook some work in Berzelius' laboratory. He became a close friend and companion of Berzelius,

travelling with him to many different countries. However, he became more and
more absorbed in his business interests and eventually abandoned his chemical
investigations altogether; the loss to science was considerable.

Arfwedson's name, like that of Svedenstjerna, was subject to some uncertainty in its spelling. It was variously rendered as 'Arfvredson' (note 21),
'Arvedson' (note 18), 'Arvidson' or 'Arfredson' (note 20); the last of these was
positively asserted, in the 1818 *Annals of Philosophy*, as being the correct
spelling, but the one used in this history is the one preferred by Johan August
himself in his writings. Berzelius, however, on a photograph of Arfwedson
which he kept in his travel diary, used the form Arfvedson.

12. Baron Jons Jacob Berzelius (1779–1848), the great Swedish scientist, has been
    justly referred to as one of the founding fathers of modern chemistry. He
    introduced the system of chemical notation by symbols, isolated selenium and
    characterised the properties of many elements (equivalents, atomic weights,
    etc.) including lithium.

13. It is not clear where the sample of petalite which Arfwedson analysed actually
    came from. It is possible that Svendenstjerna supplied it, but it could also be
    that Arfwedson, with his training in mining, obtained it himself from the island
    of Utö. Berzelius may already have possessed quantities of petalite and there is
    some evidence that he may have given samples to various colleagues, in
    addition to Arfwedson. Thus, H. G. Soderbaum in his three-volume work
    Berzelius Levnadsteckning published between 1929 and 1931 by Almqvist and
    Wiksells, Uppsala, and in his *Jac Berzelius Bref* (a collection of Berzelius'
    letters) published between 1912 and 1914, also by Almqvist and Wiksells,
    records that Berzelius was quick to communicate Arfwedson's findings to
    Wilhelm Hisinger, who was also analysing petalite, and to others, including
    Count Berthollet and Dr Marcet, who may also have been looking into the
    matter.

14. Arfwedson was a member of the editorial board of this journal, as was E. T.
    Svedenstjerna, the latter fact increasing the probability that it was from
    Svedenstjerna that Berzelius had obtained the petalite which Arfwedson used
    in his analyses. Hisinger was also on the board.

15. Arfwedson, A. (1818) 'Undersokning af nagra vid Utö Jernmalmsbrott
    forekommande Fossilier, och af ett deri funnet eget Eldfast Alkali', *Afhand-
    lingar i Fysick, Kemi och Minerologi*, 6, 145–72. The report was made available
    to a wider public when it appeared the following year, in 1819, in French
    ('Analyses de quelques minéraux de la mine d'Utö en Suède, dans lesquels on a
    trouvé un nouveau alcali fixé', *Annales de Chimie et de Physique*, 10, 82–107).

16. Vauquelin, 'Note sur une nouvelle espèce d'alcali minéral' (note 9).

17. Ibid., 284–85.

18. Clarke, E. D. (1818) 'Further account of petalite, together with the analysis of
    another new Swedish mineral found at Gryphytta, in the province of West-
    mania, in Sweden, &c.', *Annals of Philosophy*, 11, 365–68.

19. Ibid., 365.

20. Anon (1818) 'Additional observations on lithion and selenium', *Annals of
    Philosophy*, 11, 373–75. This article is actually labelled 'by Professor Berze-
    lius' but was in fact written by a member of the editorial staff of the *Annals of
    Philosophy*.

21. Thomson, T. (1818) 'History of physical science from the commencement of
    the year 1817. Part I', *Annals of Philosophy*, 12, 1–53.

22. Ibid., 16.

23. The practice of giving a single name to a compound was at that time widespread
    and only fell into eventual disuse following the introduction of Berzelius'
    symbols for the chemical elements, which paved the way for a more systematic

approach to the combination of elements. Sir Humphry Davy (see note 32) gave the names potassium and sodium to the metallic bases of potash and soda. Lithion is to lithium as potash is to potassium.

24. Gmelin, C. G. (1820) 'Analysis of petalite, and examination of the chemical properties of lithia', *Annals of Philosophy*, **15**, 341–51.
25. Clarke, 'Account of some remarkable minerals' (note 5).
26. Johann Nepomuk von Fuchs (1774–1851) was a distinguished figure in German scientific circles during the early part of the nineteenth century. A qualified medical doctor, he subsequently became a leading chemist and mineralogist, being responsible for the first definitive analyses of a number of mineral substances. He was the inventor of stereochromy, a new form of fresco painting.
27. The blowpipe was an invention of Berzelius.
28. Kobell, F. von (1857) 'Biography of Johann Nepomuk von Fuchs', *American Journal of Science*, **23**, 95–101.
29. Ibid., 99.
30. According to Jagnaux, R. (1891) *Histoire de la Chimie* (Paris: Baudry).
31. Davy probably received the lithium salt from Berzelius shortly after its preparation by Arfwedson. Although Arfwedson visited Davy in London and carried with him samples of petalite, this was in the summer of 1818 and the *Annals of Philosophy* had already carried a report in the May issue that Davy had succeeded in isolating the metallic element (see note 20).
32. Davy, H. (1807) 'The Bakerian Lecture, on some new phenomena of chemical changes produced by electricity, particularly the decomposition of the fixed alkalies, and the exhibition of new substances which constitute their bases; and on the general nature of alkaline bodies', *Philosophical Transactions*, **98**, 1–44. This long and detailed article gave accounts of Davy's isolation of sodium and potassium, but not, of course, of lithium which had yet to be discovered.
33. An anonymously written article in the 1818 *Quarterly Journal of Science and the Arts*, **5**, 337–40, gave a detailed description of Davy's lithium preparation by electrolytic means.
34. Brande, W. T. (1821) *Manual of Chemistry*, 2nd edn (London: John Murray).
35. Ibid., Vol. 2, 57.
36. Bunsen, R. and Matthieson, A. (1855) 'Dastellung des Lithiums', *Annalen der Physik und Chemie*, **94**, 107–10. In 1860, lithium was used by Bunsen in the development of the first flame spectroscope and in 1862 Robert Bunsen published the first description of lithium determination by spectroscopic means in his article, 'Über Benutzung der Flammenspektren bei der chemischen Analyse', *Verhandlungen des Naturhistorisch-medicinischen Vereins zu Heidelberg*, **2**, 31–32.

2 The first era in medicine

1. Ure, A. (1843–44) 'Observations and researches upon a new solvent for stone in the bladder', *Pharmaceutical Journal and Transactions*, **3**, 71–74.
2. Ibid., 71.
3. Ibid.
4. Lipowitz, A. (1841) 'Versuche und Resultate über die Löslichkeit der Harn-säure', *Annalen der Chemie und Pharmakologie*, **38**, 348–55.
5. Ure, 'Observations and researches upon a new solvent for stone in the bladder', 73 (note 1).
6. Ibid., 74.
7. Anon (1860) 'Calculus in the bladder, treated by litholysis, or solution of the

stone by injections of the carbonate of lithia, conjoined with lithotrity. (Under the care of Mr Ure)', *Lancet*, **ii**, 185–86. Although this article is of unascribed authorship, it is clear from the text that the greater part of it was composed by Ure himself.

8. Ibid., 186.
9. Ibid.
10. Ibid.
11. Ibid., 185.
12. Garrod, A. B. (1859) *The Nature and Treatment of Gout and Rheumatic Gout*, 1st edn (London: Walton and Maberly).
13. Ure, A. (1844–45) 'Researches on gout', *Medical Times*, **11**, 145.
14. The quotation is from Garrod, A. B. (1863) *The Nature and Treatment of Gout and Rheumatic Gout*, 2nd edn (London: Walton and Maberly) 421.
15. Garrod, A. B. (1876) *A Treatise on Gout and Rheumatic Gout (Rheumatoid Arthritis)*, 3rd edn (London: Longmans, Green and Co.) 371. Despite the change of title and publisher, this is the third edition of the book detailed in note 12.

    In relating lithium to a possible solubilising effect on uric acid, Garrod was probably much influenced by the idea put forward by Lipowitz in 1841 (see note 4) that lithium and uric acid had a special high affinity (*Verwandschaft*) for each other. Such a concept may have allowed Garrod to underplay the possibility of the low-solubility sodium urate coming out of solution in the normal *in vivo* milieu with its high sodium concentration.

16. One of the most widely used of these was Cullen, W. (1777) *First Lines of the Practice of Physic*, 1st edn (Edinburgh: W. Creech).
17. Garrod, A. B. (1883) 'The Lumleian lectures on uric acid: its physiology and its relation to renal calculi and gravel', *British Medical Journal*, **1**, 495–97.
18. Garrod's first formal statement of the possible medicinal properties of lithium seems to have been in the first edition of his book on gout. No mention was made of the matter in earlier works such as the *Elements of Materia Medica and Therapeutics* which he co-authored with E. Ballard in 1845, although in that work it was noted that mineral waters had been used in treating rheumatism and gout, where 'they act as stimulants and increase the secretion of the skin;' nor was lithium included in his 1855 work, *The Essentials of Materia Medica, Therapeutics, and the Pharmacopoeias* (London: Walton and Maberly).
19. Garrod, *The Nature and Treatment of Gout and Rheumatic Gout* (note 14).
20. Anon (1860) 'Lithium and its salts', *Chemist and Druggist*, 14 July, 241.
21. Ibid.
22. Pereira, J. (1838) *The Elements of Materia Medica and Therapeutics*, 1st edn (London: Longman, Brown, Green and Longmans). A second edition, considerably enlarged, was published four years later, in 1842. Pereira became widely known as an authority on dietary matters with the publication in 1843 of his *Treatise on Food and Diet: With Observations on the Dietetical Regimen Suited for Disordered States of the Digestive Organs; An Account of the Dietaries of Some of the Principal Metropolitan and Other Establishments for Paupers, Lunatics, Criminals, Children, the Sick, &c.* (London: Longman, Brown, Green and Longmans).
23. Lithic acid was the name originally given to uric acid by the Swedish apothecary, Karl Wilhelm Scheele in 1976.
24. Pereira, *The Elements of Materia Medica and Therapeutics*, 271 (note 22).
25. Pereira was certainly interested in alkaline substances, having written at least two articles in 1849 about chalk: 'On prepared chalk and precipitated carbonate of lime', *Pharmaceutical Journal*, **8**, 412–19; and 'Additional remarks on chalk', *Pharmaceutical Journal*, **8**, 478–80. He did not, however, record having

administered alkaline substances to any patient, with or without any medicinal end in view.

26. Cullen, *First Lines of the Practice of Physic* (note 16).
27. Garrod, *The Nature and Treatment of Gout and Rheumatic Gout* (notes 12, 14).
28. Ibid., 422.
29. Garrod, A. B. (1873) 'Renal calculus, gravel, gout and gouty deposits, and the value of lithium salts in their treatment', *Medical Times and Gazette*, 25 January, 83–84; 8 March, 246–47; and 22 March, 299–300.
30. See pp. 51–52 for further discussion of the diuretic properties of lithium salts.
31. Garrod said that he most commonly employed the carbonate and citrate of lithium, though occasionally 'for special purposes' the guaiacate was preferred.
32. Garrod, 'Renal calculus, gravel, gout and gouty deposits', 84 (note 29). To some extent this is a change of position for Garrod who, in the second edition of his text on gout, *The Nature and Treatment of Gout and Rheumatic Gout*, (note 14) had written that, 'lithia salts are of little or no avail in rheumatoid or chronic rheumatic arthritis, a disease often termed rheumatic gout; if administered in this affection their use will most probably lead to disappointment' (p. 428).
33. Garrod felt that increases in feelings of well-being were related to improvements in general health, rather than to any direct stimulant or antidepressant action of the lithium salts themselves.
34. Garrod used the term 'retrocedent gout' to refer to a malaise arising in any organ of the body following the sudden disappearance of articular affection. He felt that the organs most likely to be so affected were the stomach, intestines, heart and brain.
35. Garrod, *A Treatise on Gout and Rheumatic Gout*, 441 (note 15).
36. Ibid., 460.
37. Ibid., 461.
38. Ibid., 466.
39. Copeman, W. S. C. (1964) *A Short History of the Gout* (Berkeley and Los Angeles: University of California Press).
40. Ibid., 1.
41. Garrod, 'Renal calculus, gravel, gout and gouty deposits', 247 (note 29).
42. Garrod, *A Treatise on Gout and Rheumatic Gout*, 370 (note 15).
43. Ibid., 372.
44. The original Italian edition of Cantani's text on the pathology and treatment of metabolic disorders is not readily obtained, and all references to his ideas have been drawn from the German translation (see note 45). The Italian edition was published in 1875: Cantani, A. (1875) *Patologia e Terapia del Ricambio Materiale. Corso di Lezioni Cliniche* (Palermo: Vallardi).
45. Cantani, A. (1880) *Specielle Pathologie und Therapie der Stoffwechselkrankheiten* (Berlin: Denicke's Verlag). I am greatly indebted to Dr A. Kukopulos who has provided the details for the following brief biographic note about Cantani.

Arnoldo Cantani was born on 15 February 1837 in Hainsbach (now Lipova) between Saxony and Bohemia. He received his doctorate in medicine in 1860 in Prague. In 1868 he moved to Naples where, in 1888, he became Director of the First Medical Clinic. In 1887 he became an Italian citizen, and in 1889 he was named Senator.

As a clinician he was a positivist, and among his researches was the pathogenesis of diabetes. He explained the illness as an alteration of the metabolism of the carbohydrates, that is, as an abnormal breaking down of the sugar, caused by a particular 'ferment' contained in the pancreas, whose histological alterations in diabetes he observed and described, indicating as a therapy a diet without any food producing glucose.

Another field of his research was that of infectious illnesses. He was an enthusiastic follower of the ideas of Pasteur. In his clinic in Naples he organised the first bacteriological laboratory in Italy and the first real institute for the treatment of rabies.

He was a member of many scientific societies. He died in Naples in 1893.

46. Trousseau, A. (1868) *Clinique Médicale de l'Hôtel-Dieu de Paris*, 3rd edn (Paris: J.-B. Baillière et Fils). One of Trousseau's students, Antoine-Alphonse Gilbrin, had given a foretaste of this extension of the uric acid diathesis to encompass a variety of psychiatric syndromes, including mania (Gilbrin, A-A. (1858) *De la Diathèse Urique*. Thesis presented for the Doctorate of Medicine in the Faculty of Medicine, Paris). 'La diathèse urique porte aussi son action sur le système nerveux', he wrote, and listed 'des apoplexies nerveuses, des vertiges, de l'hypochondrie, de la manie, du délire, etc.' (pp. 14–15).

47. Trousseau, *Clinique Médicale de l'Hôtel-Dieu*, 323 (note 46). Trousseau's incorporation of 'folie' into the uric acid (gouty) diathesis became an established precept of French medicine. In 1882, Belliard summarised the cerebral concomitants of gout, amongst which he included, as well as 'folie', epilepsy, apoplexy, vertigo and hypochondria (Belliard, M. (1882) *Des Manifestations Cérébrales de la Goutte*. Thesis presented for the Doctorate in Medicine in the Faculty of Medicine, Paris).

48. The use of opium for these purposes was referred to by Cullen in 1777 in his *First Lines of the Practice of Physic* (note 16), where, writing of mania, Cullen recorded that 'according to my supposition that the disease depends upon an increased excitement of the brain, especially with respect to the animal functions, opium, so commonly powerful in inducing sleep, or a considerable collapse as to these functions, should be a powerful remedy of mania ... I have frequently employed in some maniacal cases, large doses of opium; and when they had the effect of inducing sleep, it was manifestly with advantage' (p. 62).

49. Aulde, J. (1887) 'The use of lithium bromide in combination with solution of potassium citrate', *Medical Bulletin (Philadelphia)*, **9**, 35–39; 69–72; 228–33.

50. Ibid., 38.

51. Ibid., 71.

52. Ibid.

53. Ibid.

54. Ibid.

55. Ibid., 228.

56. Ibid., 229.

57. Ibid., 230.

58. Ibid., 233.

59. Haig, A. (1892) *Uric Acid as a Factor in the Causation of Disease. A Contribution to the Pathology of High Arterial Tension, Headache, Epilepsy, Mental Depression, Gout, Rheumatism, Diabetes, Bright's, and other Disorders*, 1st edn (London: J. and A. Churchill).

60. Haig, A. (1884) 'Influence of diet on headache', *Practitioner*, **33**, 113–18.

61. Haig, A. (1886) 'Further notes on the influence of diet on headache', *Practitioner*, **37**, 179–86.

62. Ibid., 179.

63. Haig recorded the association between megrim and the uric acid diathesis as being widely accepted, but particularly so by Trousseau.

64. Dr P. W. Latham, Browning Professor of Medicine in the University of Cambridge was an acknowledged authority on the pharmacology and biochemistry of the salicylates. Haig was familiar with Latham's papers of

1885: 'Why does salicylic acid cure rheumatism?', *Lancet*, **i**, 1119–21; and 1158–60.

65. See pp. 27–28.

66. Haig, 'Further notes on the influence of diet on headache', 182 (note 61).

67. Haig, A. (1888) 'Effects in health and disease of some drugs which cause retention of uric acid, in contrast with the action of the salicylates, as shown in a previous paper', *Medico-Chirurgical Transactions*, **71**, 283–95.

68. Ibid., 289.

69. It is not certain to what uses Haig is referring, since he goes on to make it clear that he has in mind something other than Garrod's suggested use of lithium salts to treat gout.

70. Haig, 'Effects in health and disease of some drugs', 289 (note 67).

71. Haig, A. (1888) 'Mental depression and the excretion of uric acid', *Practitioner*, **41**, 342–54.

72. Ibid., 342.

73. Haig actually referred to a diurnal alternation, the uric acid blood levels being high, according to his reckoning, during the 'alkaline tide' after breakfast and again in the afternoon, and low at night when the urine showed greater acidity.

74. Haig, *Uric Acid as a Factor in the Causation of Disease*, 1st edn (note 59).

75. Haig, A. (1900) *Uric Acid as a Factor in the Causation of Disease*, 5th edn (London: J. and A. Churchill).

76. Ibid., 58.

77. The possibility of a connection between blood acidity or alkalinity and the solution of uric acid was an idea which had already been proposed in the late eighteenth century. In 1779, Dr William Hyde Wollaston in 'On gouty and urinary concretions', *Philosophical Transactions*, **87**, 386–400, had reported his studies on the solubility of concretions which he believed to consist of a mixture of substances, including lithic (uric) acid. Wollaston's work followed the assertion by Dr William Cullen in 1777 (see note 16) that both the concretions of gout, and urinary calculi, were 'very entirely' soluble in acids.

78. Haig, *Uric Acid as a Factor in the Causation of Disease*, 1st edn (note 59).

79. Murchison, C. (1874) *On the Functional Derangement of the Liver, being the Croonian Lectures* (London: Smith Elder). The Croonian Lectures were subsequently reprinted as a supplement to an altogether more detailed examination of liver dysfunction, in Murchison, C. (1877) *Chemical Lectures on the Diseases of the Liver, Jaundice and Abdominal Dropsy, Including the Croonian Lectures on Functional Derangement of the Liver, Delivered at the Royal College of Physicians in 1874.* (London: Longmans).

80. Mitchell, S. W. (1870) 'On the use of bromide of lithium', *American Journal of Medical Science*, **60**, 443–45.

81. This use of lithium bromide in the treatment of epilepsy by Mitchell (see note 80) stimulated and provided the basis of a more extensive study by Lévy: (Lévy, E. (1974) *Essai sur l'Action Physiologique et Thérapeutique du Bromure de Lithium.* Thesis presented for the Doctorate of Medicine in the Faculty of Medicine, Paris) who claimed for lithium bromide not only an anti-epileptic action, but also a more general sedative effect useful in the treatment of a variety of neurotic conditions. Lévy concluded:

> Le bromure de lithium, très-riche en brome, a une action sédative bien marquée sur l'axe cérébro-spinal. Il a modifié favorablement diverses névroses, l'épilepsie spécialement. Il est même plus actif, sous ce rapport, que le bromure de potassium. Il a encore, sur ce sel, l'avantage de ne pas agir sur le coeur et, dans un certain nombre de cas, cette propriété négative est d'un haut intérêt. On peut donc, sans crainte, promettre au bromure de lithium une place honorable dans la thérapeutique (p. 41).

The notion of lithium bromide as having therapeutic properties against some forms of epilepsy seems to have persisted well into the twentieth century. Lithium bromide was described by David Culbreth in 1927 as the 'most hypnotic of all bromides' and was recommended for epilepsy: Culbreth, D. M. R. (1927) *A Manual of Materia Medica and Pharmacology*, 7th edn (Philadelphia: Lea and Febiger). Quotation from p. 744.

82. Anon (1893) 'Effects of iodides on arterial tension excretion of urates', *Lancet*, **i**, 85–86.

83. Ibid., 86.

84. Ibid.

85. Schou, M. (1957) 'Biology and pharmacology of the lithium ion', *Pharmacological Reviews*, **9**, 17–58.

86. Lange, C. (1897) 'Bidrag til Urinsyrediatesens Klinik', *Hospitalstidende*, **5**, 1–15; 21–38; 45–63; 69–83.

    Carl Georg Lange was born in Vordingborg, Denmark on 4 December 1834. He was an intern at the Royal Frederik's and Almindelig Hospitals, Copenhagen until 1867, after which he studied physiology under Moritz Schiff in Florence for one year. He returned to Denmark to pursue studies on bulbar paralysis, cerebellar tumours, spinal meningitis, and a variety of other neuropathological topics. In 1885 he became Professor of Pathological Anatomy at the University of Copenhagen and in the same year put forward the view, which was independently promoted in the USA by the psychologist William James, that emotions resulted from awareness of the physiological reflex responses to alerting stimuli: this became known as the James–Lange theory of the emotions. Lange was a leading member of the Danish medical profession, doing much to bring awareness of major European trends in medicine to Denmark. He died in Copenhagen on 29 May 1900, aged 65. Further details of his life are to be found in Snorrason, E. (1973) 'Lange, Carl Georg'. In, Gillispie, C. C. (ed.) *Dictionary of Scientific Biography*, Vol. 8 (New York: Charles Scribner) 7–8.

87. Lange, C. (1886). *Om Periodiske Depressionstilstande og deres Patogenese*, 1st edn (Copenhagen: Jacob Lunds Forlag).

88. The correct explanation of the urinary sediment, according to Dr A. Amdisen (personal communication, 25 July 1981) was probably that the depressed patients were presenting a concentrated urine; moderate dehydration is quite common in depressed states.

89. Lange, *Om Periodiske Depressionstilstande* (note 87).

90. According to the calculations of Dr A. Amdisen (personal communication, 25 July 1981) from the dose range given in Lange's 1897 publication (note 86). Garrod, in the 1859 edition of his book on gout (note 12) recommended the use of lithium carbonate in daily doses ranging from 9 to 18 millimoles of lithium per day, whilst in the later editions of 1863 and 1876 (notes 14 and 15) the recommended daily doses lay within the broader range of 3.5 to 26 millimoles of lithium. If Lange followed Garrod's prescription, as seems likely, he will have used doses similar to those employed in the early days of lithium treatment for affective disorders.

91. Lange, C. (1896) *Periodische Depressionszustande und ihre Pathogenesis* (Hamburg and Leipzig: Verlag von Leopold Voss). The Danish version, of which the foregoing was a translation, was published the previous year: Lange, C. (1895) *Om Periodiske Depressionstilstande og deres Patogenese*, 2nd edn (Copenhagen: Jacob Lund's Forlag).

92. For example, in 1886, V. Steenberg presented a detailed critique of Carl Lange's ideas ('I Anledning af Prof. Lange's Skrift om periodiske Depressionstilstande', *Hospitalstidende*, **3**, 628–40) in which Lange's use of the uric acid

diathesis concept was greeted with particular enthusiasm: 'This observation', said Steenberg, 'is undoubtedly of such great interest that it ought to urge any doctor who treats such a patient to examine accurately, over an extended period of time, how much uric acid is excreted by these patients during the 24-hour day; so much more so because it most certainly is a question which has never been asked, and still less answered, by any psychiatric author. Prof. Lange's theory has aroused great attention among the Danish doctors and I am certain that it will not arouse less attention among doctors in other countries.' (pp. 638–39). This translation was kindly provided by Dr A. Amdisen.

Dr Knud Pontoppidan, reviewing the second Danish edition of Lange's book published in 1895, one year before the German translation (see note 91) (Pontoppodan, K. (1895) 'To psychiatriske Afhandlinger', *Hospitalstidende*, 4, 1204–10) spoke seriously of the uric acid diathesis as the basis of depression and possibly of many other psychiatric diseases.

93. Haig, *Uric Acid as a Factor in the Causation of Disease*, 5th edn (note 75).
94. Haig, 'Mental depression and the excretion of uric acid' (note 71).
95. Lange, *Om Periodiske Depressionstilstande*, 1st edn (note 87).
96. Haig, *Uric Acid as a Factor in the Causation of Disease*, 5th edn, 287 (note 75).
97. Lange C. (1895) *Om Periodiske Depressionstilstande og deres Patogenese* (Copenhagen: Jacob Lunds Forlag). This is a later and revised edition of the earlier work (note 87), all the revisions being included in an addendum summarising Lange's experiences during the intervening nine years: his sample of patients was now 2000 instead of the original 800.

In this addendum, Lange made explicit reference to Alexander Haig and to the uric acid diathesis.
98. Schou, H. I. (1938) 'Lette og begyndende Sinds-sygdomme og deres Behandling i Hjemmet', *Ugeskrift for Laeger*, **9**, 215–20.
99. Lange, *Om Periodiske Depressionstilstande*, 1st edn (note 87).
100. I am indebted to Dr A. Amdisen for providing a translation of the appropriate phrase from H. I. Schou's article (note 98). 'Behandling af Depression bestaar i Isolation og Sengeleje. Det var en Misforstaaelse, naar Carl Lange tidligere strabaserede disse Patienter for at tjerne den "urinsure Diatese", som ikke findes' (p. 217); that is, 'The treatment of depression consists of isolation and confinement to bed. It was a misunderstanding when Carl Lange earlier exercised [lit. 'over-worked'] these patients to remove the "uric acid diathesis" which does not exist'. And, of course, if the uric acid diathesis did not exist, nor did the justification for using lithium as a treatment for depression.

One should mention, however, that H. I. Schou made his comments not with endogenous depression *in general* in mind, but with specific reference to the slight and 'masked' depressions described by Lange and to which H. I. Schou proposed the label 'depression mentis sine depressione'.
101. Lange, F. (1894) *De vigtigste Sindssygdomsgrupper*, (Copenhagen: Gyldendalske Boghandels Forlag). This book did have some impact within Denmark, and in 1896 F. Lange's views about the use of lithium in treating depression were made a central theme in an article by F. Levison (Levison, F. (1896) 'Om Depressionstilstandes forhold til Urinsyre', *Hospitalstidende*, 4, 353–84) in which he rejected the views of Garrod and C. Lange on the aetiology of gout and instead suggested that urates might be deposited round the joints and in the kidneys, at which latter point they irritated and stimulated neural reflex arcs to other organs, thereby eliciting all the symptoms subsumed under the uric acid diathesis (Garrod's 'irregular gout') including depression. Levison indicated that orally administered lithium carbonate, by dissolving the urates, stopped the reflex arc stimulation and hence alleviated depression.
102. Gibb, G. D. (1865) 'Note on the action of the bromides of lithium, zinc and

lead', *Reports of the 34th Meeting of the British Association for the Advancement of Science*, 123.

103. Ibid.
104. Ibid.
105. See p. 15.
106. Mitchell, 'On the use of bromide of lithium', 443 (note 80).
107. A number of requests for personal reminiscences, documents, etc., related to the history of lithium treatment were inserted in a variety of medical journals in 1980 and 1981; these drew some interesting responses, and material from the communications received is incorporated into the text at various points.
108. This was in 1955 – it was clearly still thought that the lithium citrate was inhibiting kidney stone formation.
109. Anon (1981), personal communication.
110. Soranus of Ephesus (AD 98–138) studied medicine at Alexandria and became a practitioner of medicine in Rome under the Emperors Trajan and Hadrian. Only one of his works still exists, the *Gynaecia* (which is concerned exclusively with obstetrical and gynaecological matters), but his writings were widely translated, abridged and excerpted, surviving in that form to exert a powerful influence on medical practice and thought up to the Middle Ages.
111. Caelius Aurelianus was the most important of the translators of Soranus' writings, and of these translations the treatises upon acute diseases and chronic diseases are the most important and first appeared in printed form in 1529 (*De Morbis Acutis et Chronicis*) in an edition by Johannes Sichart and published in Basel by Heinricht Petri.
112. According to Soranus, natural (mineral) waters were suitable for a bewildering range of conditions. The following list is taken from the edited translation of Caelius Aurelianus' *On Acute Diseases and Chronic Diseases* provided by I. E. Drabkin (1950) (University of Chicago Press).

Condition	Comments
Chronic headache	Bathing in the waters.
Epilepsy	Bathing in the waters.
Mania	'Use should be made of natural waters, such as alkaline springs, particularly those free from any pungent odour' (p. 553). It is not clear from this whether bathing or drinking is implied, but from the context it would seem that bathing is more likely.
Paralysis	Bathing.
Earache	Drinking might be implied, but it is more probable that Soranus is suggesting that the water should be poured into the ear.
Toothache	As a mouth wash.
Catarrh	Probably the inhalation of vapours.
Diseases of the oesophagus	Drinking is clearly intended here, in addition to bathing: 'it is well also to prescribe the use of natural springs, for instance, the Cutilian and the Nepesine in Italy; have the patient bathe in these waters and drink them, for this will be most beneficial' (p. 739).
Diseases of the liver and spleen	Inhalation of vapours.
Jaundice	Bathing.
Cachexia	Bathing.
Failure of nutrition	Bathing.
Dropsy	Warmth from the vapours.

Elephantiasis	(Probably a form of leprosy) Bathing.
Coeliac disease	Bathing.
Diseases of the colon	Bathing and probably also drinking.
Arthritis and podagra	It is not clear what is implied; drinking the waters may be involved, but bathing seems more likely.
Diseases of the bladder	Swimming is specifically recommended, but 'in cases of bladder stone or scabies, choose waters containing salt or nitrum, e.g. the springs on the island of Aenaria; these springs should be used for both drinking and bathing' (pp. 955 and 957).
Internal abscesses	Drinking probably.
Obesity	Bathing.

113. In 1568, William Turner, then Dean of Wells, published a book entitled *A Booke of the Natures and Properties as well as of the Bathes in England as of other Bathes in Germanye and Italye etc.* (London); this was a survey of the therapeutic benefits to be derived from mineral springs, and had originally been written as an appendix to a book on English medicinal plants, published in 1592. A review has recently appeared of the history of mineral water therapy in seventeenth-century English medicine (Coley, N. G. (1979) 'Cures without care: "Chymical physicians" and mineral waters in seventeenth-century English medicine', *Medical History*, **23**, 191–214). In this article, the writer records that the warm-water springs at Bath and Buxton, after being well-known to the Romans, fell into decline during the Middle Ages, to become once again of interest towards the end of the sixteenth century, particularly for the treatment of rheumatism, gout, and diseases of the skin. This revival of the fortunes of Bath and Buxton was chronicled by John Jones in 1572 (*The Benefit of the Ancient Bathes of Buckstones which Cureth most Grievous Sicknesses, never before Published*, and *The Bathes of Bathe Ayde*, both published in London); it quickly became widespread intelligence that these waters were of benefit against bladder stones and gravel.

114. It is of course true that, whatever the medical benefits to be gained from the waters, the congenial nature of hydropathic treatment, particularly in attractive settings, made it very popular with the more wealthy members of society who, in their turn, were thus inclined to accept and encourage a notion, such as that stemming from the uric acid diathesis concept, of a single treatment for a range of symptoms and diseases. To be fair to the physicians of the time, they were not unaware that much of the therapeutic efficacy apparently possessed by the mineral springs was perhaps more accurately ascribed to the congenial surroundings in which the waters were taken. Dr Willard H. Morse ((1887) 'A contribution to the study of the therapy of lithia water', *The Medical Age*, **5**, 433–34), after writing ecstatically about lithia, which he claimed to be 'possessed of certain peculiar advantages, which render it the best exponent of akaline therapeutics' (p. 433), agreed that there were other, less easily determined, factors involved, such as 'physical influences of change of scene and associations' (p. 434). He went on to remark that 'excellent though the water is as found in the market, seven-fold better are the draughts taken from the springs as it bubbles forth glad with granitic flavours' (p. 434).

115. Ibid.

116. Ibid., 433.

117. Ibid., 434.

118. Ibid.

119. Cruise, F. R. (1885) 'Notes of visits to Contrexéville and Royat-les-Bains', *Lancet*, **i**, 1121–23.

120. Ibid., 1123.
121. See p. 26.
122. Cruise, 'Notes of visits to Contrexéville and Royat-les-Bains' (note 119).
123. Cruise, F. R. (1885) 'Notes of visits to Contrexéville and Royat-les-Baines', *Lancet*, **i**, 1160–1161, quotation from 1160.
124. Emond, E. (1885) 'On the treatment of bronchial asthma at Mont Dore, France', *Lancet*, **i**, 1161–63.
125. Ibid., 1161.
126. A report of this work by Berzelius appeared in English two years later: Anon (1826) 'Prof. Berzelius's discovery of lithia in mineral waters', *Annals of Philosophy*, **11**, 145–46.
127. Osann, E. (1839) *Physikalisch-Medicinische Darstellung der bekannten Heilquellen der vorzuglischsten Lander Europa's* (Berlin: Ferdinand Dummler.)
128. Ure, 'Observations and researches upon a new solvent for stone in the bladder', 71 (note 1).
129. Yeo I. B. (1888) 'An address on the therapeutics of the uric acid diathesis, delivered at the opening of a discussion on the subject in the Section of Pharmacology and Therapeutics at the Annual Meeting of the British Medical Association, held in Dublin, August, 1887', *British Medical Journal*, **1**, 16–19 and 67–72.
130. Yeo, I. B. (1893) *A Manual of Medical Treatment or Clinical Therapeutics* (London: Cassell and Co.).

   A much fuller account was later given in Yeo, I. B. (1904) *The Therapeutics of Mineral Springs and Climates* (London: Cassell and Co.). In this volume, Yeo refers to the mineral springs at Neuenahr in Germany, Obersalzbrunn in Silesia, Fachingen, Bilin and Assmannshausen, and notes that these springs are especially rich in lithium. He goes on to say that these waters stimulate free diuresis and may be beneficial in the treatment of conditions related to the gouty diathesis. In the period between Yeo's 1893 and 1904 works a considerable amount of analytical work was carried out on the mineral waters of Europe, much of this being summarised by Perrandeau in Perrandeau, H. (1898) *Essai sur l'Action Thérapeutique du Carbonate de Lithine et de l'Eau Lithinée dans la Diathèse Goutteuse*. Thesis presented for the Doctorate of Medicine in the Faculty of Medicine, Paris. In view of the results of later analyses which showed just how little lithium the mineral waters actually contained, the analyses summarised by Perrandeau clearly owed more to the eye of faith than to analytical accuracy.
131. James, F. L. (1889) 'Lithium in mineral waters', *St Louis Medical and Surgical Journal*, **57**, 24–30.
132. In the first place, the imperial gallon was used in quoting concentrations, whilst the American standard gallon was the unit of sale: this resulted in a 20 per cent inflation of the lithium content. Secondly, the figures related to the crystalline and not the anhydrous form of the salt, a device which could lead to overestimation of the salt by as much as 100 per cent.
133. Waller, E. (1890) 'Determination of lithia in mineral waters', *Journal of the American Chemical Society*, **12**, 214–23.
134. Harrington, C. (1896) 'On the action of commercial lithia waters', *Boston Medical and Surgical Journal*, **135**, 644–45.
135. Ibid., 645.
136. Leffmann, H. (1910) 'Lithia waters as therapeutic agents', *Monthly Cyclopaedia and Medical Bulletin, Philadelphia*, **3**, 138–44.
137. Quoted by Strobusch, A. D. and Jefferson, J. W. (1980) 'The checkered history of lithium in medicine', *Pharmacy in History*, **22**, 72–76. There were many such judgments made in courts of law. Tuckahoe Lithia Water, a product of the

Tuckahoe Mineral Springs Company, Pennsylvania, which was described by the company as 'a sure solvent for calculi, either of the kidneys or liver' was declared, in a legal judgment, to be misbranded. Londonderry Lithia Water, sold by a New Hampshire spring water company for 'Rheumatism, Neuralgia, Dyspepsia, Eczema, Malarial Poisoning, Gout, Gravel, Bright's Disease, Diabetes, Dropsy, and all diseases of the Kidneys and Bladder' had so little lithium in it that to obtain any reasonable dose, a person would, according to evidence presented in court, have to consume considerably more than 225 barrels of the water. These judgments were recorded in the *Journal of the American Medical Association* and were included in an edited collection of such items: Cramp, A. J. (1921) *Nostrums and Quackery: Articles on the Nostrum Evil and Quackery Reprinted from the Journal of the American Medical Association.* Vol. 2 (Chicago: American Medical Association Press).

138. James, 'Lithium in mineral waters', 25 (note 131).
139. Harrington, 'On the action of commercial lithia waters', 644 (note 134).
140. Leffmann, 'Lithia waters as therapeutic agents', 144 (note 136).
141. According to Leffmann, (note 136) 'excellent distilled waters can now be obtained at moderate cost and druggists can easily dissolve a small amount, say five grains, of the pure carbonate in a gallon and the water can be used as desired in place of ordinary drinking water' (p. 144).
142. Strobusch and Jefferson, 'The checkered history of lithium in medicine' (note 137).
143. Anon (1908) 'Lithia water', *Chemist and Druggist*, 31 October, 681–82.
144. Ibid., 682.
145. Thuillier, J. (1981) *Les Dix Ans qui ont Changé la Folie* (Paris: Opera Mundi).
146. Ibid., 261–62.
147. Anon (1880) 'medicated lozenges', *Chemist and Druggist*, 15 December, 516.
148. Yeo, 'An address on the therapeutics of the uric acid diathesis' (note 129).
149. Ibid., 68.
150. Jahns (1883) *Archiv der Pharmakologie*, **21**, 7. Quoted by Good, C. A. (1903) 'An experimental study of lithium', *American Journal of Medical Science*, **125**, 273–84.
151. Krumhoff (1884) *Wirkung des Lithium*. Inaugural dissertation (Gottingen). Quoted by Good, in 'An experimental study of lithium' (note 150).
152. Anon (1860) 'Lithium and its salts', *Chemist and Druggist*, 14 July, 241.
153. Ibid.
154. Siebold, L. (1889) 'Medical and chemical misconceptions about lithia, *Chemist and Druggist*, 14 September, 367–68.
155. Ibid., 368.
156. Anon (1894) 'The value of lithium salts', *Chemist and Druggist*, 29 September, 490.
157. Ibid.
158. Porteus, J. L. (1893) 'The therapeutics and treatment of the uric acid diathesis', *New York Medical Journal*, **55**, 71–73.
159. Ibid., 71.
160. Ibid.
161. Ibid.
162. Ibid., 72.
163. Kolipinski, L. (1898) 'Notes on some toxic effects from the use of citrate of lithium tablets', *Maryland Medical Journal*, **40**, 4–5.
164. Strandgaard, N. J. (1899) *Gigt: og Urinsur Diatese* (Copenhagen: Jacobs Lunds Medicinske Boghandel).
165. *Larousse Medical Illustré* (1912) (Paris: Librairie Larousse).
166. Ibid., 30.

167. The association of tuberculous joint infection and other varieties of arthritic disorder is, indeed, of long standing. Copeman, in his *A Short History of the Gout* (note 39), records that both Hippocrates and Soranus of Ephesus gave accounts of arthritic complaints which corresponded closely to the modern view of tubercular infection, and that as late as 1909 a condition referred to as 'tuberculous rheumatism' was proposed by Professor Poncet who supposed that a tuberculous infection carried in the blood might give rise, in certain cases, to a generalised rheumatoid arthritis.

It is also pertinent to note that Garrod, in the third edition of his treatise on gout (note 15), reported the employment of the bark of the common ash tree in the treatment of scrofulous and gouty affections, and the use, by the peasants of the Auvergne, of ash leaves as a remedy for gout: the association between scrofula and gout, and the subsuming of both under the single heading of the uric acid diathesis would, therefore, not have been unnatural.

168. Moitessier, M. J. (1903) 'Influence des sels de lithium sur la solubilité de l'acide urique et des urates', *Comptes Rendus des Séances de la Société de Biologie (Paris)*, **55**, 1032–33.

169. Daniels, A. L. (1914) 'The influence of lithium and atophan on the uric acid excretion of a gouty patient', *Archives of Internal Medicine*, **13**, 480–84.

170. Ibid., 484. Evidence to support Haig's view that lithium would reduce, rather than increase, uric acid output, was provided by E. W. Rockwood and C. Van Epps (1907) 'The influence of some medicinal agents on the elimination of uric acid and creatinine', *American Journal of Physiology*, **19**, 97–107.

171. Weiss, H. (1924) 'Ueber eine neue Behandlungsmethode des Diabetes mellitus und Verwandter Stoffwechselstorungen', *Weiner Klinische Wochenschrift*, **37**, 1142 and 1263.

172. Isaac, S. (1924) 'Ueber Lithizit bei Diabetes', *Wiener Klinische Wochenschrift*, **37**, 1263.

173. Depisch, F. (1924) 'Ueber eine neue Behandlungsmethode des Diabetes mellitus und Verwandter Stoffwechselstorungen', *Wiener Klinische Wochenschrift*, **37**, 1216.

174. Morse, 'A contribution to the study of the therapy of lithia water' (note 114).

175. Garrod, *The Nature and Treatment of Gout and Rheumatic Gout*, (note 12).

176. Dyson, M. (1931) 'The alkali metals in chemistry and pharmacy: III. The compounds of lithium, rubidium and caesium', *Pharmaceutical Journal and Pharmacist*, **127**, 202–04.

177. Ibid., 204. The same scepticism was also expressed by A. Beuer (1932) 'Die biologische Wirkung der Lithiumsalze und ihre therapeutische Verwendbarkeit', *Schweizerische Medizinische Wochenschrift*, **13**, 135–40.

178. Mercier, J. (1947) 'Action de deux sels organiques de lithium sur la diathèse et l'élimination de l'acide urique chez le lapin', *Comptes Rendus des Séances de la Société de Biologie (Paris)*, **141**, 491–94. Some years earlier, a series of fairly detailed studies carried out in Italy had reaffirmed a possible uricolytic effect of lithium salts: Spoto, P. (1930) 'Ricerche sui farmaci uricolitii. Nota I: I sali di litio', *Archivio di Scienze Biologiche (Bologna)*, **15**, 324–41.

179. Zollner, N. (1957) *Thanhausers Lehrbuch des Stoffwechsels und der Stoffwechselkrankheiten* (Berlin: Georg Thieme Verlag). The idea of a possible solubilising action of lithium salts on uric acid seems, indeed, to have been particularly resilient in Germany culminating in 1964 in a study by Arne-Andreas Kollwitz, 'Zur therapeutischen Verwendbarkeit von Lithium salzen beim Harnsäuresteinleiden', *Der Urologe*, **3**, 360–63, in which the kidneys of dogs were perfused with lithium chloride, but without effect on renal calculi. Kollwitz concluded that lithium treatment for kidney stones was no longer indicated.

180. Hazard, R. (1956) *Précis de Thérapeutique et de Pharmacologie* (Masson:

Paris). To be fair, Hazard did add the comment that 'leur action dissolvante est beaucoup moins nette en présence de chlorure de sodium et d'autres sels de l'urine, car c'est alors l'urate le moins soluble qui a tendance à se former; aussi leur action *in vivo* est-elle très douteuse'.

181. Talbott, J. H. (1964) *Gout*, 2nd edn (New York: Grune and Stratton). The first edition appeared in March 1943.

182. Ibid., 12.

183. Martindale, W. (1883) *The Extra Pharmacopoeia of Unofficial Drugs and Chemical and Pharmaceutical Preparations*, 1st edn (London: H. K. Lewis).

184. Mitchell, 'On the use of bromide of lithium' (note 80).

185. Martindale, W. (1884) *The Extra Pharmacopoeia of Unofficial Drugs and Chemical and Pharmaceutical Preparations*, 2nd edn (London: H. K. Lewis).

186. Ibid., 170.

187. Martindale, W. (1885) *The Extra Pharmacopoeia with Additions Introduced into the British Pharmacopoeia, 1885*, 4th edn (London: H. K. Lewis).

188. Ibid., 229.

189. Ibid.

190. Garrod, *The Nature and Treatment of Gout and Rheumatic Gout*, (note 12).

191. Yeo, 'An address on the therapeutics of the uric acid diathesis' (note 129).

192. Martindale, W. (1888) *The Extra Pharmacopoeia with Additions Introduced into the British Pharmacopoeia, 1885*, 5th edn (London: H. K. Lewis).

193. Ibid., 241.

194. Garrod, 'Renal calculus, gravel, gout and gouty deposits' (note 29).

195. Ibid., 299. It is also worth noting that, in 1887, there appeared the third edition of T. Lauder Brunton's *Textbook of Pharmacology, Therapeutics and Materia Medica* (London: Macmillan) and in this widely-read and influential text the doctrine of lithium-induced solubility of body urates was repeated, with particular reference being made to the topical administration of lithium salts. According to Brunton, lithia 'is applied locally to parts affected with gouty inflammation ... It may be applied to stiff joints and chalk-stones, whether covered by the skin or laid bare by ulceration. A solution of lithia ... is kept constantly applied to the part for several weeks altogether' (p. 632).

196. Huffner, Von. G. (1881) 'Ueber die Undurchlassigkeit der menschlichen Haut für Losungen von Lithionsalz', *Zeitschrift für Physiologische Chemie*, **4**, 378–81.

197. See note 64.

198. T. Lauder Brunton, in his *Textbook of Pharmacology* (note 194), made the point quite explicitly. Lithium salicylate, he said 'is intended to unite the properties of salicylic acid and lithium' (p. 633). It should, however, be noted that, even in 1888, at the time of the fifth edition of the *Extra Pharmacopoeia*, there was already considerable dispute about the efficacy of the salicylates in treating gout.

199. Garrod, 'The Lumleian lectures on uric acid' (note 17).

200 Hippuric acid was so named because of having first been discovered in the urine of horses.

201. Martindale, W. (1895) *The Extra Pharmacopoeia*, 8th edn (London: H. K. Lewis).

202. Ibid., 281.

203. Ibid.

204. Ibid.

205. Mendelsohn, M. (1893) 'Zur Therapie der harnsäuren Diathese', *Verhandlung des Congresses für innere Medicin: Zwölfter Congress* (Wiesbaden: J. F. Bergman).

206. Martindale, W. (1898) *The Extra Pharmacopoeia Revised in Accordance with the "British Pharmacopoeia", 1898*, 9th edn (London: H. K. Lewis).

207. Ibid., 23.
208. Ibid., 298.
209. Martindale, W. and Westcott, J. W. (1901) *The Extra Pharmacopoeia*, 10th edn (London: H. K. Lewis).
210. Ibid., 319.
211. Martindale, W. H. and Westcott, W. W. (1904) *The Extra Pharmacopoeia of Martindale and Westcott*, 11th edn (London: H. K. Lewis).
212. Martindale, W. H. and Westcott, W. W. (1906) *The Extra Pharmacopoeia of Martindale and Westcott*, 12th edn (London: H. K. Lewis).
213. Ibid., 460.
214. Yeo, 'An address on the therapeutics of the uric acid diathesis' (note 129).
215. Ibid., 68.
216. See pp. 27–28.
217. Martindale, W. H. and Westcott, W. W. (1908) *The Extra Pharmacopoeia of Martindale and Westcott*, 13th edn (London: H. K. Lewis).
218. Ibid., 113.
219. Martindale, W. H. and Westcott, W. W. (1910) *The Extra Pharmacopoeia of Martindale and Westcott*, 14th edn (London: H. K. Lewis).
220. Martindale, W. H. and Westcott, W. W. (1915) *The Extra Pharmacopoeia of Martindale and Westcott*, 16th edn (London: H. K. Lewis).
221. See pp. 46–7.
222. Martindale, W. H. and Westcott, W. W. (1922) *The Extra Pharmacopoeia of Martindale and Westcott*, 17th edn (London: H. K. Lewis).
223. Martindale, W. H. and Westcott, W. W. (1924) *The Extra Pharmacopoeia of Martindale and Westcott*, 18th edn (London: H. K. Lewis).
224. Ibid., 357.
225. Ibid., 242.
226. Ibid.
227. *The Extra Pharmacopoeia: Martindale* (1941) 22nd edn (London: The Pharmaceutical Press).
228. Ibid., 678.
229. Blacow, N. W. (ed.) (1972) *Martindale. The Extra Pharmacopoeia, Incorporating Squire's Companion*, 26th edn (London: The Pharmaceutical Press).
230. *Merck's Index* (1889) 1st edn.
231. *Merck's Index* (1907) 3rd edn.
232. *Merck's Index* (1930) 4th edn.
233. *The Merck Index* (1940) 5th edn.
234. *The Merck Index* (1952) 6th edn.
235. *The Merck Index* (1960) 7th edn.
236. *The Merck Index* (1968) 8th edn.
237. *The Merck Index* (1976) 9th edn.
238. Martindale and Westcott, *The Extra Pharmacopoeia*, 14th edn (note 219).
239. Amdisen, A. (1981). Personal communication, 3 March.
240. Ibid.
241. The calculations are those provided by Dr Amdisen, ibid.
242. Ibid.
243. Ohlendorf, D. (1981). Personal communication, 23 November.
244. Dr Ohlendorf, Pharmacy Director of the Universitätsklinikum Charlottenburg, in the Free University of Berlin, kindly compiled a complete list of lithium-containing preparations currently available in West Germany (see note 243).
    Dr Ricardo Bach, of Bach Associates Incorporated, South Carolina, has also provided details of a preparation called Togal® which is available as a controlled, but over-the-counter, drug in West Germany. The composition of Togal® is:

Quinine hydrochloride	1.5 mg
Acetyl salicylic acid	250.0 mg
Lithium citrate	42.0 mg
Binding agent	40.0 mg

A 333.3 mg tablet contains 3.6 mg of lithium, that is about 1.08 per cent. Togal® is prescribed in the accompanying literature as an antirheumatic agent and is described as being used for pain in joints and limbs, headaches, migraine and 'under-the-weather' feelings; it is also remarked that 'rheumatism and neuralgias are a closely related group of illnesses which show changes in tissues: Togal® fundamentally affects these pathological processes by stimulating uric acid exchange'. I am indebted to Dr Bach for providing this translation.

245. An advertisement for the varalettes appeared in the *Chemist and Druggist Diary* (1933) 95.
246. Amdisen, A. (1981). Personal communication, 27 October. The full details of the composition of the lithium benzoate-containing preparation were given in the Finnish publication *Pharmaka* (1940) 497.
247. See p. 19.
248. Amdisen, personal communication, (note 246).
249. Hes, J. Ph. (1980). Personal communication, 25 December.
250. Anumonye, A., Reading, H. W., Knight, F. and Ashcroft, G. W. (1968) 'Uric acid metabolism in manic–depressive illness and during lithium therapy', *Lancet*, **i**, 1290–93.

3 The work of John Cade

1. Cade, J. F. J. (1980). Personal communication, 12 August.
2. Ibid.
3. Cade, J. Jr. (1981). Personal communication, 18 May.
4. Ibid.
5. Cade, J. F. J. (1970) 'The story of lithium'. In, Ayd, F. J. *Discoveries in Biological Psychiatry* (Philadelphia: Lippincott) 218–29.
6. Ibid., 220.
7. Cade, J. F. J. (1978) 'Lithium – past, present and future'. In, Johnson, F. N. and Johnson, S. *Lithium in Medical Practice* (Lancaster: MTP Press) 5–16.
8. Ibid.
9. Ibid., 12.
10. Cade, J. F. J. (1949) 'Lithium salts in the treatment of psychotic excitement', *Medical Journal of Australia*, **36**, 349–52.
11. Ibid.
12. Cade, 'Lithium – past, present and future', 12 (note 7).
13. Nathan Kline produced one of the early historical surveys of lithium therapy: Kline, N. S. (1969) 'Lithium: the history of its use in psychiatry', *Modern Problems in Pharmacopsychiatry*, **3**, 75–92.
14. Kline, N. S. (1973) 'A narrative account of lithium usage in psychiatry'. In, Gershon, S. and Shopsin, B. *Lithium: Its Role in Psychiatric Research and Treatment* (New York: Plenum Press) 10.
15. Good, C. A. (1903) 'An experimental study of lithium', *American Journal of Medical Science*, **125**, 273–84.
16. Cleaveland, S. A. (1913) 'A case of poisoning by lithium presenting some new features', *Journal of the American Medical Association*, **60**, 722.
17. See pp. 46–57.
18. Cade, J. F. J. (1967) 'Lithium in psychiatry: historical origins and present position', *Australian and New Zealand Journal of Psychiatry*, **1**, 61–62.

19. Cade, J. Jr., personal communication, (note 3).
20. Cade, 'Lithium salts in the treatment of psychotic excitement', 8 (note 10).
21. Cade, J. F. J., personal communication, (note 1). In several of his later articles, Cade referred to 'that august publication, the *British Pharmacopoeia*' (see, for example, note 7, p. 15).
22. Cade, J. F. J., personal communication, (note 1).
23. Cade, 'Lithium salts in the treatment of psychotic excitement' (note 10).
24. Ibid., 352.
25. Ibid., 350.
26. The original cards bearing Cade's case notes are now in the Medical History Museum of the University of Melbourne, Australia. I am grateful to Professor Brian Davies of the Department of Psychiatry at Melbourne University for sending me photographs of the cards, and to Professor Attwood of the Medical History Museum for giving his permission for extracts from the notes to be used in this book.
27. Original case notes of J. F. J. Cade, 8 February 1950.
28. Ibid., 12 May 1950.
29. See p. 40.
30. This observation is interesting in the light of the uric acid diathesis which had held sway in medicine prior to this time (see Chapter 2).
31. Original case notes, 6 March 1949.
32. Cade, 'Lithium salts in the treatment of psychotic excitement', 351 (note 10).
33. Original case notes, 21 February 1950.
34. Cade, 'Lithium salts in the treatment of psychotic excitement', 351 (note 10).
35. Original case notes, 1 March 1949.
36. Ibid., 5 March 1949.
37. Ibid., 10 April 1949.
38. Cade, 'Lithium salts in the treatment of psychotic excitement' (note 10).
39. Ibid., 351.
40. Original case notes, 4 March 1949.
41. Ibid., 10 March 1949.
42. Ibid., 15 March 1949.
43. Ibid., 8 February 1950. In the case notes the date was actually recorded as 8 January, but this would appear to have been an error, since the preceding entry in the notes was dated 20 January.
44. Ibid., 2 March 1950.
45. Ibid., 3 May 1950.
46. Ibid., 12 May 1950.
47. Ibid., 19 May 1950.
48. Ibid., 22 May 1950.
49. Ibid., 23 May 1950.
50. Ibid.
51. Cade, 'Lithium salts in the treatment of psychotic excitement', 351 (note 10).
52. Gershon, S. and Yuwiler, A. (1960) 'Lithium ion: a specific psychophar-macological approach to the treatment of mania', *Journal of Neuropsychiatry*, **1**, 229–41.
53. Cade, J. F. J., personal communication, (note 1).
54. Cade, J. F. J. (1969) 'The use of lithium salts in the treatment of mania', *Supplement to the Bulletin of the Post-Graduate Committee in Medicine, University of Sydney*, **25**, 528–33.
55. Ibid., 530.
56. For example, Ronald Fieve (1975) in his remarkable book *Moodswing: The Third Revolution in Psychiatry* (New York: Morrow) says: 'His [John Cade's] discovery of lithium's antimanic effect was entirely serendipitous' (p. 248).

57. Cade, 'Lithium – past, present and future', 9–10 (note 7).
58. These studies were outlined in Cade, 'The story of lithium' (note 5).
59. Ibid., 225.
60. Ibid., 228.
61. The first coincidence was referred to in Chapter 2 (p. 17).
62. I am indebted to Mr W. Chick, Deputy Hospital Administrator at the Mid-Wales Hospital, Talgarth, Brecon, Wales, for providing me with details of Dr Jones' appointment to Victoria.
63. Dr Diggle (see note 64) was aware that the manufacturers of the lithium salt, Messrs Ferris and Company of Bristol, had changed the style of their labels around that time, and he recalled that the canister carried a label of the old style. Unfortunately, it is not possible to confirm that Ferris and Co. actually did supply lithium to the Mid-Wales Hospital around the turn of the century, since all records except those of essential manufacturing processes were destroyed during the Second World War, according to Mr P. J. Jenks, Assistant Manager to the company (Personal communication, 8 February 1982).
64. Diggle, G. (1981). Personal communication, 3 November.
65. Dr Ernest Jones became a figure of some influence in psychiatry, and a clinic named after him exists at the present time in the Royal Melbourne Hospital (Davies, B. (1982). Personal communication, 5 January). Jones was Cade's immediate predecessor in the Victoria Department of Mental Hygiene, though Dr E. Cunningham Dax, who joined the department in 1951 (Personal communication from Dr Dax to Professor Brian Davies, 27 January 1982) doubts that Jones knew Cade well since, on the dozen or so occasions that Dax and Jones met, Jones never mentioned Cade, though the work of the department was actually discussed a great deal.

    In none of Jones' published writings is lithium therapy once mentioned.
66. Amdisen, A. (1981). Personal communication, 15 September.
67. Debbie Guthridge of the Royal Melbourne Hospital Pharmacy Department's Drug Information Service, has provided a survey of lithium availability in Australia.
68. It was only in 1968 that lithium was included in the appropriate schedule of the 1962 Poisons Act in Australia, and thereby became restricted to a doctor's prescription; prior to that time, a wide variety of lithium preparations was available over the counter, subject only to the pharmacist's discretion.
69. John Cade would not, I think, have been averse to being described as a 'rediscoverer'; he often thought of himself in such terms, and took, indeed, a measure of pride in undertaking investigations which led him – perhaps by a different route – to conclusions previously reached by other investigators. Examples of this are given in my obituary notice of John Cade, published in 1981: 'John F. J. Cade, 1912 to 1980: a reminiscence', *Pharmacopsychiatria*, **14**, 148–49. Professor Mogens Schou of Aarhus University, Denmark, has also made this point very nicely (Schou, M. (1977). After-dinner speech in honour of John Cade. Melbourne, 4 February 1977). Schou referred to a visit which John Cade and his wife Jean had made to Aarhus:

    I wanted to show them a bit of our country. It is nice but not spectacular, so we chose to show them something that was old. We first took them to a neolithic stone monument, and John became very interested. He started measuring angles, sighting along stone edges, and asking where north was. He wanted to find out whether perhaps this Danish monument, like the 2000 years younger Stonehenge in England, had served the function of an astronomy observatory. I am afraid Jean, Nete and I pulled him away before he had completed his observations.

We next went to see two medieval churches in Aarhus, the Cathedral and the Church of Our Lady. The latter is distinguished by having a crypt church, that is a small older church under the floor of the choir. The occurrence of a crypt church is infrequent although not rare, but this particular one was interesting by having been hidden and forgotten for many centuries. Only twenty tears ago it was found by accident and turned out to be the oldest existing church in Scandinavia, dating from about AD 900. The story of this discovery excited John, and when he was again up in the main church, he started to go over its floor systematically stamping on each individual stone slab and listening. He wanted to see whether perhaps yet another crypt church could be hidden under the floor.

These two incidents told me something about the man and the scientist: The insatiable curiosity, the keen observation, the willingness to test even the absurdly unlikely hypothesis, the courage to run the risk of making a fool of himself. This is the stuff innovators are made of – and of course fools. John's contribution has not been foolish.

70. Cade, J. F. J. (1979) *Mending the Mind* (Melbourne: Sun Books).
71. Dr J. L. Evans, one of Cade's colleagues, drew attention to this fact in a graceful obituary which he wrote about John Cade in the *Medical Journal of Australia*, 2 May 1981, 489; referring to 'the characteristic modesty which allowed him to write the pages about the discovery of lithium treatment without revealing that he was personally responsible'.

4   The toxicity panic

1. Full historical details of the introduction of psychoactive drugs into psychiatry are to be found in Ban, T. A. (1969) *Psychopharmacology* (Baltimore: Williams and Wilking Co.).
2. Leake, C. D. (1958) *The Amphetamines* (Springfield: Charles C. Thomas).
3. Ban, *Psychopharmacology* (note 1).
4. John Cade was not slow to claim this status for lithium treatment. Reviewing his work in his paper 'Lithium in psychiatry: historical orgins and present position', *Australian and New Zealand Journal of Psychiatry*, 1, 61–62, he said: 'There are few specifics in medicine. The specific antimanic effect of the lithium ion is one of them' (p. 61).
5. See Chapter 5.
6. *The Extra Pharmacopoeia: Martindale* (1936) 21st edn (London: The Pharmaceutical Press).
7. Also sold as Wes-sal, this was the first lithium-containing salt substitute to be put on the market.
8. The precise composition of Westsal was given by the American Medical Association Chemical Laboratory as:

lithium chloride	25.0	per cent
citric acid	0.2	per cent
potassium iodide	0.01	per cent
water	74.79	per cent

according to an editorial note in the 12 March 1949 edition of the *Journal of the American Medical Association*, 692.
9. Anon (1949) 'Case of the substitute salt', *Time*, 28 February, 27. By permission of *Time* magazine, the weekly news magazine © Time Inc. 1949.
10. A footnote inserted at this point in the original report gave the following details: Foods Plus Inc, Manhattan, makers of Foodsal; Lueth's Bakery, Kansas City, makers of Salti-salt.

11. Anon, 'Case of the substitute salt' (note 9).
12. Ibid.
13. Hanlon, L. W., Romaine, M. III., Gilroy, F. J. and Deitrick, J. E. (1949) 'Lithium chloride as a substitute for sodium chloride in the diet. Observations on its toxicity,' *Journal of the American Medical Association*, **139**, 688–92.
14. Radomski, J. L., Fuyat, H. N., Nelson, A. A. and Smith, P. K. (1950) 'The toxic effects, excretion and distribution of lithium chloride', *Journal of Pharmacology and Experimental Therapeutics*, **100**, 429–44.
15. Anon, 'Case of the substitute salt' (note 9).
16. Waldron, A. M. (1949) 'Lithium intoxication', *Journal of the American Medical Association*, **139**, 733. This was actually a preliminary communication; a longer and more detailed report was published elsewhere: Waldron, A. M. (1949) 'Lithium intoxication', *University Hospital Bulletin*, **15**, 9–10.
17. Hanlon *et al.*, 'Lithium chloride as a substitute for sodium chloride in the diet' (note 13).
18. Waldron, 'Lithium intoxication', *Journal of the American Medical Association* (note 16).
19. Anon, 'Case of the substitute salt' (note 9).
20. Ibid.
21. Corcoran, A. C., Taylor, R. D. and Page, I. H. (1949) 'Lithium poisoning from the use of salt substitutes', *Journal of the American Medical Association*, **139**, 685–88. Dr G. Masson contributed an Addendum to this report in which he described similar toxic reactions in rats. This may well have helped to convince the readers that the deaths were actually due to lithium and not to the illnesses of the patients (both of whom were, in any case, elderly and suffering from arteriosclerotic heart disease).
22. Stern, R. L. (1949) 'Severe lithium chloride poisoning with complete recovery. Report of a case', *Journal of the American Medical Association*, **139**, 710–11.
23. The FDA statement to this effect was issued on 18 February 1949.
24. Statement issued by the FDA on 18 February 1949 and quoted in Aaron, H. (1949) 'Dangerous drugs', *Consumer Reports*, **14**, 171–73.
25. Issued on 28 February 1949.
26. Issued on 2 March 1949; quoted in Aaron, 'Dangerous drugs', 172 (note 24).
27. Ibid.
28. The results of the studies were published later in Radomski *et al.* 'The toxic effects, excretion and distribution of lithium chloride' (note 14).
29. Aaron, 'Dangerous drugs', 173 (note 24).
30. Anon (1860) 'Caclulus in the bladder, treated by litholysis, or solution of the stone by injections of the carbonate of lithia, conjoined with lithotrity. (Under the care of Mr Ure)', *Lancet*, **ii**, 185–86.
31. Gibb, G. D. (1865) 'Note on the action of bromides of lithium, zinc and lead', *Reports of the 34th Meeting of the British Association for the Advancement of Science*, 123.
32. Garrod, A. B. (1873) 'Renal calculus, gravel, gout and gouty deposits, and the value of lithium salts in their treatment', *Medical Times and Gazette*, 25 January, 83–84; 8 March, 246–47; and 22 March, 299–300.
33. Garrod, A. B. (1876) *A Treatise on Gout and Rheumatic Gout (Rheumatoid Arthritis)*, 3rd edn (London: Longmans, Green and Co.).
34. Ibid., 370.
35. Garrod, A. B. (1859) *The Nature and Treatment of Gout*, 1st edn (London: Walton and Maberly).
36. Garrod, *A Treatise on Gout and Rheumatic Gout* (note 33).
37. Ibid., 370.
38. For example, in 1876, Dr A. Hesse made reference to Garrod in this context, in

his doctoral dissertation entitled *Lithion*, presented to the Medical Faculty of Göttingen.

39. Rambuteau (1868) *Études Expérimentales sur les Effets Physiologiques des Florures et des Composés Métalliques en Générale* (Paris: Germer Baillière). Quoted in Good, C. A. (1903) 'An experimental study of lithium', *American Journal of Medical Science*, **125**, 273–84.

40. Quoted in Good, 'An experimental study of lithium' (note 39). He gives as his reference only 'California Academy of Sciences'.

41. Hesse, *Lithion* (note 38). In connection with the use of lithium to treat phenomena supposedly related to the uric acid diathesis, a variety of side effects were quite well known around the time that Hesse was writing. For example, two years earlier, in 1874, Climent (Climent, E. (1874). *Traitement de la Gravelle Urique*. Thesis presented for the Doctorate of Medicine in the Faculty of Medicine, Paris) wrote: 'Sur ce point, nous pouvons nous prononcer catégoriquement. Nous l'avons experimenté, et nous avons vu qu'à la dose de 2 grammes (comme M. Charcot l'a donné), il nous a été impossible de le supporter plus de quatre jours. Il a provoqué chez nous l'apparition de troubles dyspeptiques que nous n'avions jamais éprouvés antérieusement. Ces manifestations gastriques se produiront donc toujours et d'autant mieux chez les graveleux et les goutteux, qui sont généralement, avant tout, dyspeptiques' (p. 33).

42. Brunton, T. L. and Cash, J. T. (1884) 'Contributions to our knowledge of the connexion between chemical constitution, physiological action, and antagonism', *Philosophical Transactions of the Royal Society*, **175**, 197–244. Good, 'An experimental study of lithium' (note 39), quoted this article, but his reference to it was completely wrong: indeed, the accuracy and appropriateness of the references given by Good are of a generally low standard.

43. Krumhoff (1884) *Wirkung des Lithium*. Inaugural Dissertation, Göttingen. Quoted by Good, 'An experimental study of lithium' (note 39).

44. Richet, C. (1886) 'De l'action physiologique des sels alcalins. Études de toxicologie générale', *Archives de Physiologie Normale et Pathologique*, **7**, 101–50.

45. Binet, P. (1892) 'Sur la toxicité comparée des métaux alcalins et alcalino-terreux', *Comptes Rendus des Séances de l'Académie des Sciences (Paris)*, **115**, 251–53.

46. See pp. 20–23.

47. Kolipinski, L. (1898) 'Note on some toxic effects from the use of citrate of lithium tablets', *Maryland Medical Journal*, **40**, 4–5.

48. Good, 'An experimental study of lithium' (note 39).

49. Luff, A. P. (1907) 'The treatment of some of the forms of gout', *The Practitioner*, **68**, 161–75.

50. Ibid., 166–67. This report was quoted by John Cade in many of his writings, though Cade never managed to get the reference quite right. It is, perhaps, worth pointing out that if Cade actually ever read Luff's paper he would have been aware of the use of lithium in treating what were referred to as the 'irregular' forms of gout, including insomnia – a condition often associated with mood disturbance.

51. Cleaveland, S. A. (1913) 'A case of poisoning by lithium, presenting some new features', *Journal of the American Medical Association*, **60**, 722.

52. Good, 'An experimental study of lithium' (note 39).

53. Cleaveland, 'A case of poisoning by lithium' (note 51).

54. There were occasional references to a diuretic effect (Menzani, G. (1934) 'Il litio e il ricambio dei metalli alcalin ed alclino terrosi', *Archivio Italiano di*

Scienze e Farmacologia, **3**, 45–58) and to the lethal dose levels in various animals (Alles, G. A. and Knoeffel, P. K. (1939) 'Comparative physiological actions of alkyl-trimethylammonium and of alkali-metal salts', *University of California Publications in Pharmacology*, **1**, 187–211; and Simonin, P. and Pierron, A. (1947) 'Toxicité brute des derivés fluores', *Comptes Rendus des Séances de la Société de Biologie, Paris*, **124**, 133–34. In the 1940s a few references appeared to a possible influence of lithium salts on embryonic development in sea urchins (Needham, J. (1942) *Biochemistry and Morphogenesis* (Cambridge University Press); and Lehmann, F. E. (1945) *Einfurung in die physiologische Embryologie* (Basel: Birkhauser Verlag)) and in chicks (Naz, J. F. and Rulon, O. (1946) 'Modification of development in the chick with LiCl and NaCNS', *Anatomical Record*, **96**, 555) but since by this time lithium salts were not being used therapeutically on any scale, the findings evoked no reactions from the medical world.

55. Aaron, 'Dangerous drugs' (note 24).
56. Peters, H. A. (1949) 'Lithium intoxication producing chorea athetosis with recovery', *Wisconsin Medical Journal*, **48**, 1075–76.
57. Greenfield, I., Zuger, M., Bleak, R. M. and Bakal, S. F. (1950) 'Lithium chloride intoxication', *New York State Journal of Medicine*, **50**, 459–60.
58. For example: Leusen, I. and Demeester, G. (1950) 'Au sujet de la toxicité du chlorure de lithium', *Acta Medica Scandinavica*, **138**, 232–36; Davenport, V. D. (1950) 'Distribution of parenterally administered lithium in plasma, brain and muscle of rats', *American Journal of Physiology*, **163**, 633–41; and Radomski, J. L., Fuyat, H. N., Nelson, A. A. and Smith, P. K. (1950) 'The toxic effects, excretion and distribution of lithium chloride', *Journal of Pharmacology and Experimental Therapeutics*, **100**, 429–44.
59. Roberts, E. L. (1950) 'A case of chronic mania treated with lithium citrate and terminating fatally', *Medical Journal of Australia*, **37**, 261–62.
60. Ashburner, J. V. (1950) 'A case of chronic mania treated with lithium citrate and terminating fatally', *Medical Journal of Australia*, **37**, 386.
61. Ibid.
62. Talbott, J. H. (1950) 'Use of lithium salts as a substitute for sodium chloride', *Archives of Internal Medicine*, **85**, 1–10.
63. This is the constitution of Westsal and, although Talbott at no point identifies it as such, it is clear from the description which he gives of the panic over lithium toxicity, that it was indeed Westsal that he was investigating.
64. The average daily intake by patients allowed unrestricted use of the salt substitute was 0.5 g of lithium chloride per day. In his studies involving higher dose levels, Talbott increased this to between 2.0 g and 5.0 g per day.
65. Talbott, 'Use of lithium salts as a substitute for sodium chloride', 4 (note 62).
66. Ibid., 5.
67. This value is, of course, well in excess of what would normally be regarded as a safe level in modern lithium therapy, though there are some psychiatrists who have advocated high dose levels where these are necessary to produce a therapeutic response.
68. Talbott, 'Use of lithium salts as a substitute for sodium chloride', 7–8 (note 62).
69. Ibid., 9.
70. Soloff, L. A. and Zatuchni, J. (1949) 'Syndrome of salt depletion induced by a regimen of sodium restriction and sodium diuresis', *Journal of the American Medical Association*, **139**, 1136–39.
71. Ibid., 1139.
72. This point had been made, though less forcefully, in many of the earlier reports of toxicity.

5 Early confirmations

1. See Chapter 2.
2. Young, R. M. (1980). Personal communication, 23 October.
3. The correct reference was: Cade, J. F. J. (1949) 'Lithium salts in the treatment of psychotic excitement', *Medical Journal of Australia*, **36**, 349–52.
4. Dr Young (note 2) added a footnote to his letter concerning this point:

> I have just discovered a reference in my father's Hale White's *Materia Medica* of 1899, recommending lithium, including effervescent citrate, for the treatment of gout because of the solubility in lithium urate but casting doubt on its effectiveness *in vivo*. No doubt my bottle of lithium citrate was a relic of that era.

5. Ashburner, J. V. (1950) 'A case of chronic mania treated with lithium citrate and terminating fatally', *Medical Journal of Australia*, **37**, 386.
6. Cade, 'Lithium salts in the treatment of psychotic excitement' (note 3).
7. Ashburner, J. V. (1982). Personal communication, 4 March.
8. E. M. Trautner is an interesting figure in the history of lithium therapy, but few of the published historical sketches make more than a passing mention of the man or his work. Professor R. Douglas Wright, of the Howard Florey Institute of Experimental Physiology and Medicine, University of Melbourne, Australia, has kindly provided a brief sketch of Trautner's life (Wright, R. D. (1981). Personal communication, 26 August) in which he records that Trautner, a Berliner by birth, fell foul of the Nazi party as a result of a book which he wrote implicating the Nazis in a political murder, and was forced to flee to England in 1933 just before the Nazi party came to power. Shortly after the commencement of the war, Trautner was deported to Australia, along with his common-law wife, Jill, and her two children. In Australia, Trautner sought release from internment, joining Douglas Wright's Department of Physiology at Melbourne University on 17 August 1942, where he became involved in developing procedures for extracting pharmaceutical products from plants. After the war Trautner went back briefly to England, to the School of Botany at Oxford, and then returned to join Wright in Melbourne to carry out investigations on nervous tissue metabolism, and later became involved with work on lithium. Trautner left the Department of Physiology at Melbourne on 31 December 1961 and retired to the warmer climate of Queensland, having persuaded his companion, Jill, to change her name by deed-poll to Trautner thereby saving, as Trautner told it, a lot of money by avoiding costly divorce proceedings. He died in 1976. Jill died four years later.
9. Professor V. Wynn is currently Director of the Alexander Simpson Laboratory for Metabolic Research at St Mary's Hospital Medical School, University of London.
10. Wynn, V. (1982). Conversation, 21 September.
11. Wynn, V., Simon, S., Morris, R. J. H., McDonald, I. R. and Denton, D. A. (1950) 'The clinical significance of sodium and potassium analyses of biological fluids: their estimation by flame spectrophotometry', *Medical Journal of Australia*, **37**, 821–36.
12. R. H. Morris, who was also working with the team investigating sodium and potassium, recalls Trautner's enthusiasm for arranging serum estimations (Morris, R. H. (1981). Personal communication, 11 September).

> I was a recently married postgraduate and took a day off to start a new lawn at home. My work involved flame-photometric analysis of sodium and

potassium in connection with studies on ion-binding to cell constituents, and it so happened that on that day Trautie assured Charlie Noack who was then in the Department of Mental Hygiene and interested in feeding lithium to manic–depressives, that it would be no trouble to me to run a few lithium samples through for him. I forget how many thousand samples I finally did during the period.

13. Noack, C. H. and Trautner, E. M. (1951) 'The lithium treatment of maniacal psychosis', *Medical Journal of Australia*, **38**, 219–22.

14. Ibid., 222.

15. Talbott, J. H. (1950) 'Use of lithium salts as substitutes for sodium chloride', *Archives of Internal Medicine*, **85**, 1–10.

16. See pp. 46–57.

17. Noack and Trautner's article was remarkable in a number of ways. In particular, it foreshadowed much later work on patterns of lithium excretion related to clinical response.

18. Despinoy, M. and Romeuf, J. de (1951) 'Emploi des sels de lithium en thérapeutique clinique', *Comptes Rendus du Congrès des Médécins Alienistes et Neurologistes de Langue Française, (Rennes)*, 509–15;
Reyss-Brion, R. and Grambert, J. (1951) 'Essai de traitment des états d'excitation psychotique par le citrate de lithium', *Journal de Médécine de Lyon*, **32**, 985–89;
Deschamps and Denis [no initials were given in the original article] (1952) 'Premiers résultats du traitement des états d'excitation maniaque par les sels de lithium', *L'Avenir Medical (Lyon)*, **49**, 673–79;
Duc, N. and Maurel, H. (1953) 'Le traitement des états d'agitation psychomotrice par le lithium', *Concours Médical*, **75**, 1817–20 (this was also reported in abstract form: Lafon R., Duc, N. and Maurel, H. (1953) 'Traitement des états d'excitation psychomotrice par le carbonate de lithium', *Presse Médical*, **61**, 713);
Carrère, J. and Pochard Mlle [no initials were given for Mlle Pochard] (1954) 'Le citrate de lithium dans le traitement des syndromes d'excitation psychomotrice', *Annales Médico-Psychologiques*, **112**, 566–72;
Plichet, A. (1954) 'Le traitement des états maniaques par les sels de lithium', *Presse Médical*, **62**, 869–70;
Sivadon, P. and Chanoit, P. (1955) 'L'emploi du lithium dans l'agitation psychomotrice à propos d'une expérience clinique', *Annales Médico-Psychologiques*, **113**, 790–96;
Teulie, Follin and Begoin [no initials were given] (1955) 'Étude de l'action des sels de lithium dans états d'excitation psychomotrice', *Encéphale*, **44**, 266–85;
Oulès, J., Soubrie, R. and Salles, P. (1955) 'À propos du traitement des crises de manie par les sels de lithium', *Comptes Rendus du Congrès des Médécins Alienistes et Neurologistes de Langue Française*, 570–73;
Oulès, J. (1955) 'Discussion', *Annales Médico-Psychologiques*, **113**, 679.

To these published reports one might also add a doctoral thesis produced in Paris in 1955: Maissin, C. M-T. L. P. (1955) *Le Traitement de la Manie par le Citrate de Lithium*. Thesis presented for the Doctorate of Medicine in the Faculty of Medicine, Paris. In this, a number of cases were described of the successful treatment of mania by lithium citrate, the author concluding that 'au total, nous pouvons dire que le citrate de lithium nous semble être, actuellement, le meilleur traitement de la manie' (p. 48). It is also of interest, in view of the later prophylactic uses of lithium, that Maissin recommended long-term administration of lithium: 'Nous insistons, en effet, sur l'importance de *prolonger ce traitement* d'entretien en raison du fait que l'arrêt de la thérapeutique entraine une rechute rapide du malade' (p. 47).

19. Giustino, P. (1953) 'Il citrato di litio nel trattamento degli stati di eccitazione psicotica', *Note e Riviste di Psichiatria (Pesaro)*, **79**, 307–11.
20. Noack and Trautner, 'The lithium treatment of maniacal psychosis' (note 13); Glesinger, B. (1954) 'Evaluation of lithium in treatment of psychotic excitement', *Medical Journal of Australia*, **41**, 277–83;
    Margulies, M. (1955) 'Suggestions for the treatment of schizophrenic and manic–depressive patients', *Medical Journal of Australia*, **42**, 137–41;
    Trautner, E. M., Morris, R., Noack, C. H. and Gershon, S. (1955) 'The excretion and retention of ingested lithium and its effect on the ionic balance of man', *Medical Journal of Australia*, **42**, 280–91.
21. Schou, M., Juel-Nielsen, N., Strömgren, E. and Voldby, H. (1954) 'The treatment of manic psychoses by the administration of lithium salts', *Journal of Neurology, Neurosurgery and Psychiatry*, **17**, 250–60;
    Schou, M., Juel-Nielsen, N., Strömgren, E. and Voldby, H. (1955) 'Behandling af maniske psykoser med lithium', *Ugeskrift for Laeger*, **117**, 93–101.
22. Reyss-Brion and Grambert, 'Essai de traitment des états d'excitation psychotique par le citrate de lithium', 988 (note 18).
23. Duc and Maurel, 'Le traitment des états d'agitation psychomotrice par le lithium' (note 18).
24. Guistino, 'Il citrato di litio nel trattamento degli stati...' (note 19).
25. For example, Daumezon, G., Guibert, M. and Chanoit, P. (1955) 'Un cas d'intoxication grave par le lithium', *Annales Médico-Psychologiques*, **113**, 673–79.
26. Trautner *et al.*, 'The excretion and retention of ingested lithium' (note 20).
27. Dr Gershon is currently Director of the Lafayette Clinic, Detroit and Chairman and Professor of Psychiatry at Wayne State School of Medicine, Detroit, Michigan.
28. Gershon, S. (1980). Personal communication, 16 October.
29. Wright, personal communication (note 8).
30. Ashburner, J. V. (1981). Personal communication, 15 June.
31. See pp. 95–96.
32. Trautner *et al.*, 'The excretion and retention of ingested lithium' (note 20).
33. Ibid., 281.
34. Glesinger, B., 'Evaluation of lithium in treatment' (note 20).
35. Ibid., 280.
36. Ibid., 282.
37. Schou, M. *et al.*, 'The treatment of manic psychoses by the administration of lithium salts' (note 21).

6 Beginning of the second era in medicine

1. Professor Schou has written about the early history of lithium therapy research at Aarhus: Schou, M. (1979) 'Lithium research at the Psychopharmacology Research Unit, Risskov, Denmark: A historical account'. In, Schou, M. and Strömgren, E. (eds) *Origin, Prevention and Treatment of Affective Disorders* (London: Academic Press) 1–8.
2. Ibid., 1.
3. See pp. 15–17.
4. Strömgren, E. (1980). Personal communication, 2 October.
5. See p. 17.
6. Schou, M. (1957) 'Biology and pharmacology of the lithium ion', *Pharmacological Reviews*, **9**, 17–58.
7. Schou, M. (1981). Personal communication, 4 January.

8. See pp. 94–96.

9. Schou refers to the review of the history of lithium therapy compiled by Nathan Kline: Kline, N. S. (1969) 'Lithium: the history of its use in psychiatry', *Modern Problems of Pharmacopsychiatry*, **3**, 75–92.

10. Schou, Personal communication (note 7).

11. Schou, 'Lithium research at the Psychopharmacology Research Unit', 1 (note 1). It was not, of course, the first such trial in medicine. Schou (conversation, 18 March 1982) has noted that it might have been the influence of Rolv Gjessing's work on periodic catatonia which had provided the main inspiration for the first lithium trial: Schou had spent some three months working with Gjessing.

12. Schou, M., Juel-Nielsen, N., Strömgren, E. and Voldby, H. (1954) 'The treatment of manic psychoses by the administration of lithium salts', *Journal of Neurology, Neurosurgery and Psychiatry*, **17**, 250–60.

13. Noack, C. H. and Trautner, E. M. (1951) 'The lithium treatment of maniacal psychosis', *Medical Journal of Australia*, **38**, 219–22. This article was also cited by Rice (Rice, D. (1956) 'The use of lithium salts in the treatment of manic states', *Journal of Mental Science*, **102**, 604–11) as being the stimulus for his own work, which was the first to be published in England. Schou wrote to Trautner in 1974 and expressed his opinion that Trautner's work had played a seminal role in lithium therapy:

   I still remember clearly the correspondence we had in the early fifties, and it is my firm conviction that the studies you contributed concerning lithium toxicity and the monitoring of lithium treatment through serum lithium determinations were of primary importance for the development of this treatment into a safe and efficient procedure. Much has happened to lithium since then, but we are still taking advantage of your contributions (Schou, M. (1974). Letter to E. M. Trautner, 27 November).

14. In the light of what is now known about lithium intoxication, it seems likely that the death may have been hastened, if not actually precipitated, by the very high serum lithium levels in this patient.

15. Schou, *et al.*, 'The treatment of manic psychoses by the administration of lithium salts', 254 (note 12).

16. Schou, M., Juel-Nielsen, N., Strömgren, E. and Voldby, H. (1955) 'Behandling af maniske psykoser med lithium', *Ugeskrift for Laeger*, **117**, 93–101.

17. Reported by Schou, M. (1959) 'Lithium in psychiatric therapy: stock-taking after ten years', *Psychopharmacologia*, **1**, 65–78.

18. Sivadon, P. and Chanoit, P. (1955) 'L'emploi du lithium dans l'agitation psychomotrice à propos d'une expérience clinique', *Annales Médico-Psychologiques*, **113**, 790–96; Teulie, Follin and Begoin [no initials given] (1955) 'Étude de l'action des sels de lithium dans états d'excitation psychomotrice', *Encéphale*, **44**, 266–85. The stimulus for the French work is unclear. Schou was not contacted by any of the groups of French investigators at the time.

19. Gershon, S. and Trautner, E. M. (1956) 'The treatment of shock-dependency by pharmacological agents', *Medical Journal of Australia*, **43**, 783–87.

20. Noack and Trautner, 'The lithium treatment of maniacal psychosis' (note 13).

21. Rice, D. (1956) 'The use of lithium salts in the treatment of manic states', (note 13).

22. Andreani, G., Caselli, G. and Martelli, G. (1958) 'Rilievi clinici ed elettro-encefalografici durante il trattamento con sali di litio in malati psichiatrici', *Giornal di Psichiatria e Neuropatologia*, **86**, 273–328.

23. Schou, 'Lithium in psychiatric therapy: stock-taking after ten years' (note 17), referred to observations made by Belling, but still in press in 1955; the report

was not actually published until four years later: Belling, G. (1959) 'Lithium-behandling på et sindssygehospital', *Ugeskrift for Laeger*, **121**, 1193–95.

24. Schou, 'Lithium in psychiatric therapy: stock-taking after ten years' (note 17), included in his survey all cases of typical mania together with less typical ones in which manic symptoms predominated; both chronic and acute cases were listed, and hypomanic as well as true manic cases. Schou did not include any cases in which there was a major psychotic component in addition to mania, or in which the lithium had been applied purely prophylactically or after a preliminary electroshock treatment.

25. These further results have been noted by Kline, 'Lithium: the history of its use in psychiatry' (note 9), and include data from groups in France, the Soviet Union, Italy and Czechoslovakia.

26. One should, perhaps, interpret with some caution the reports referred to in note 25, since in most cases the criteria for assessing clinical improvements were not clear, and it is by no means certain that all the patients fell within the diagnostic limits applied by Schou in his stock-taking review of 1959 (note 17).

27. Schou, 'Lithium research at the Psychopharmacology Research Unit' (note 1).

28. Ibid., 2.

29. Schou, M. (1958) 'Lithium studies. 1. Toxicity', *Acta Pharmacologica et Toxicologica*, **15**, 70–84; Schou, M. (1958) 'Lithium studies. 2. Renal elimination', *Acta Pharmacologica et Toxicologica*, **15**, 85–98; Schou, M. (1958) 'Lithium studies. 3. Distribution between serum and tissues', *Acta Pharmacologica et Toxicologica*, **15**, 115–24.

30. Schou, M. (1982). Conversation, 18 March.

31. Masson, G. (1949) 'Addendum', *Journal of the American Medical Association*, **139**, 688.

32. Corcoran, A. C., Taylor, R. D. and Page, I. H. (1949) 'Lithium poisoning from the use of salt substitutes', *Journal of the American Medical Association*, **139**, 685–88.

33. Schou, et al., 'Behandling af maniske psykoser med lithium' (note 16).

34. Dr Baastrup has kindly provided a copy of the text of his talk given to the staff meeting at his hospital in April 1960. The text is in Danish, but Dr Baastrup's English translation is presented below:

> Altogether there are fifty-six patients, diagnostically a rather heterogeneous group with the common symptom of exaltation. The diagnosis for the largest group is manic–depressive psychosis with most of the patients in the manic phase and a few in the depressive. The other conditions are psychogenic exultation, exulted phases of paranoia or schizophrenia, and, lastly, chronic psychotic patients who have been manic for shorter or longer periods.
>
> During the time we have tried it at this hospital, the use of lithium has largely been experimental, and the duration of treatment has therefore been inadequate in a number of cases. Treatment has been stopped owing to intoxication symptoms, and, for a while, we may have allowed a single, very severe case of intoxication to alarm us. Treatment has also been discontinued because it had no immediate effect on the psychotic condition, patients may have been unstable, have refused to take the tablets, or stopped taking them after discharge. We may have used lithium too much as a therapeutic agent and too little as a prophylactic.

35. Baastrup, P. C. (1980). Personal communication, 21 November.

36. Ibid.

37. Baastrup, P. C. (1964) 'The use of lithium in manic–depressive psychosis', *Comprehensive Psychiatry*, **5**, 396–408.

38. Dr G. P. (Toby) Hartigan was born on 12 August 1917. At the time of his work

on lithium prophylaxis he was Deputy Medical Superintendent and Consultant Psychiatrist at St Augustine's Hospital, Chartham Down, and Consultant Psychiatrist to the Kent and Canterbury Hospital. Dr J. A. Ainslie, who was Medical Superintendent at St Augustine's, remembers Hartigan as a highly intelligent, witty individual, 'and I think he might reasonably have been described as a bon viveur' (Ainslie, J. A. (1982). Personal communication, 29 March). An intimate insight into his personality is provided by his wife, Mrs Elizabeth Hartigan.

> Only on rare occasions did Toby bring work, or problems, home. He was more likely to ask me to read some observations he intended putting to the Cricket Committee, or a letter of praise or criticism, usually the latter to Mr Raymond Postgate, in the early days of the *Good Food Guide*. Their correspondence was amusing, sometimes hilarious and frequently in sloughs of despair, but encouraging to each other. Basically Toby was an investigator, in his work and in his hobbies, a 'lister' and indexer, cross-references his forte. These could be on Popes, music, churches, pictures, wines, restaurants – but not gardening. He encouraged me in my gardening efforts, but on the whole, he preferred it wild, which it usually was.
>   Holidays were planned with enormous care. I recall a trip we made to Venice. Toby had the walks we should take typed out several months ahead, and in fact arriving, as we did, at 4.00 a.m. the first walk was knocked off before breakfast. But this holiday produced an exciting find for him. On the last day but one, with the itinerary completed, we took an unscheduled trip to, to his mind and the guide book's, a meritless church on the outskirts of Venice. It was dull, but nearby was a public loo, unnumbered. I didn't know that every building in Venice had a number, even the loos. He was quite gleeful over this find. I often wonder if he wrote to the Venetian authorities, which he might have done with an element of devilment, but also, of course, the map was not complete without this vital number. He was fastidious about detail for himself, but forgiving of those who found it irksome or unimportant. (Hartigan, E. (1982). Personal communication, 26 April.)

Toby Hartigan died suddenly on 28 June 1968, of a massive coronary. He was 50.

39. The number was given as eight by Schou in a later report (Schou, M. (1963) 'Normothymotics, "mood-normalizers": are lithium and imipramine drugs specific for affective disorders?', *British Journal of Psychiatry*, **109**, 803–09), but Hartigan's text for his 1959 presentation indicates that there were seven patients with recurrent depressions.
40. A brief summary of the talk appeared two years later: Hartigan, G. P. (1961) 'Experiences of treatment with lithium salts,' *Journal of Mental Science*, Suppl., 49.
41. Schou, *et al.*, 'The treatment of manic psychoses by the administration of lithium salts' (note 12).
42. Hartigan, G. P. (1960). Letter to M. Schou, 29 August.
43. Schou, M. (1960). Letter to G. P. Hartigan, 7 September.
44. Ibid.
45. Schou, conversation (note 30).
46. Schou, M. (1961). Letter to G. P. Hartigan, 16 November.
47. Schou's account of this visit was reported in Johnson, F. N. and Cade, J. F. J. (1975) 'The historical background to lithium research and therapy'. In, Johnson, F. N. (ed.) *Lithium Research and Therapy* (London: Academic Press) 9–22.

48. Schou, M. (1962). Letter to G. P. Hartigan, 27 February.
49. Ibid.
50. Schou, conversation (note 30).
51. Schou, M. (1962). Letter to G. P. Hartigan, 11 September.
52. Ibid.
53. Hartigan, G. P. (1962). Letter to M. Schou, 17 September.
54. Hartigan, G. P. (1962). Letter to M. Schou, 24 October.
55. Ibid.
56. Hartigan (1962). Letter to M. Schou, 18 December.
57. Hartigan, G. P. (1963) 'The use of lithium salts in affective disorders', *British Journal of Psychiatry*, **109**, 810–14.
58. Baastrup, P. C. (1981). Personal communication, 5 November.
59. Baastrup, 'The use of lithium in manic–depressive psychosis' (note 37). Baastrup's paper was, in fact, prepared well in advance of its actual publication date. In 1963 Schou ('Normothymotic, "mood-normalizers"', note 39) made a reference to Baastrup's findings, noting that Baastrup had 'used lithium with slightly different indications: in patients with mixed (transitional) manic–depressive psychosis and in cases with very frequent and rapid changes between manic and depressive phases' (p. 806) and whilst some forty of these patients failed to respond, 'in 12 cases lithium was accompanied by a normalisation, by a prevention of not only the manic but also the depressive attacks'. This information was referenced in the text as 'Baastrup (1962)' but appears in the bibliographic list as 'Baastrup (1963). To be published'.
60. Schou, (conversation, note 30), felt that it would be appropriate for Baastrup and Hartigan to publish their accounts separately and independently since this most accurately represented the nature of the discovery, and also because Schou felt that two reports of the same finding would be likely to have a greater impact than a single combined report.
61. Schou, 'Normothymotics, "mood-normalizers"' (note 39).
62. A word derived from *norma* (Latin = 'normal') and *thymos* (Greek = 'mind' or 'spirit', particularly the affective component). The term never really caught on in psychiatry – a fact which might be mainly due to its ugliness, but which is in any case the just desert of a term with such bastard linguistic origins. A further suggestion that drugs might be classified as 'symptomolytics' or 'nosolytics' was also mercifully passed over.
63. The Third International Collegium Neuropsychiatricum.
64. The rationale for Schou's paper on normothymotics was first spelled out in detail in a letter which he sent to Hartigan in 1962 (note 48).
65. Schou, (conversation, note 30) has expressed the opinion that his decision to submit his 'normothymotics' paper for publication may have been a mistake, on the grounds that his views about lithium and imipramine were still ill formed, and their public airing premature. Certainly the style of the article differs from his others: it is much more speculative and provocative. Nevertheless, there is no doubt that it did arouse interest in lithium, and highlighted a problem – the classification of lithium amongst other psychiatric drugs – which still causes considerable confusion and about which there exists no clear consensus even today.
66. Schou, M. (1961). Letter to G. P. Hartigan, 31 August.
67. Ibid.
68. Hartigan, G. P. (1961). Letter to M. Schou, 2 September.
69. Schou, M. (1981). Address on receiving an honorary doctorate. University of Aix-Marseille, 29 October.
70. Baastrup, P. C. and Schou, M. (1967) 'Lithium as a prophylactic agent: its effect against recurrent depression and manic–depressive psychosis', *Archives*

of General Psychiatry, **16**, 162–72. This work had been presented the previous year (1966) at a meeting in Madrid, Spain, of the World Psychiatric Congress. It took the form of a brief article in *Sandorama* (a journal issued by the pharmaceutical company Sandoz): Schou, M. and Baastrup, P. C. (1966) 'Lithium and manic–depressive psychosis', *Sandorama*, Special number, 48–49.

71. Baastrup and Schou, 'Lithium as a prophylactic agent', 162 (note 70). The collaboration between Baastrup and Schou was (and remains) a particularly happy one though they worked, and work, in different hospitals in different parts of Denmark (Baastrup at the Psychiatric Hospital in Glostrup and Schou at the Psychiatric Hospital in Aarhus, Risskov). The personal styles of the two differed in ways which interacted to produce a most fruitful result. Baastrup was the cautious collector of data, disinclined either to speculate too strongly about the possible implications of his results or to move too quickly to publication. Schou provided the organising influence: more used to expressing himself in English than was Baastrup, Schou set about the task of presenting the clinical data in the most meaningful way, and of seeing to their publication.

72. In a letter to Angst (Schou, M. (1983). Personal communication to J. Angst, 6 January) Schou recalled the start of the collaborative effort:

> We first discussed lithium prophylaxis at the Meeting in Haiti in April 1966. I remember clearly that on the first day of the meeting I told about prophylaxis in the morning, and at the lunch, given by the Minister of Health, we sat opposite each other at the table, and we discussed whether we might perhaps join forces, since you had information on the disease course and also patient material that might be well suited for prophylactic studies . . .
>
> Our collaborative study started in 1967, and it was in December 1968 that we submitted our paper to the Anna-Monika Foundation. I remember vividly my winter visit to Zurich and our hectic activity to finish the paper before the deadline of 31 December 1967.

73. Angst, J., Dittrich, A. and Grof, P. (1969) 'Course of endogenous affective psychoses and its modification by prophylactic administration of imipramine and lithium', *International Pharmacopsychiatry*, **2**, 1–11. This article was first delivered as a communication to the Royal Medico-Psychological Association at its Annual Meeting in Plymouth, England, 12 July 1968.

74. Ibid., 3.

75. Angst, J., Weis, P., Grof, P., Baastrup, P. C., and Schou, M. (1970) 'Lithium prophylaxis in recurrent affective disorders', *British Journal of Psychiatry*, **116**, 604–14. In fact, the collaboration went beyond simply trying to establish clinical efficacy. Practicalities of therapy were also considered, as for example in Schou, M., Baastrup, P. C., Grof, P., Weis, P. and Angst, A. (1970) 'Pharmacological and clinical problems of lithium prophylaxis', *British Journal of Psychiatry*, **116**, 615–19. A third article to come out of the Anna-Monika report dealt with methodological issues: Grof, P., Schou, M., Angst, J., Baastrup, P. C. and Weis, P. (1970) 'Methodological problems of prophylactic trials in recurrent affective disorders', *British Journal of Psychiatry*, **116**, 599–603.

76. Kline, 'Lithium: the history of its use in psychiatry' (note 9).

77. Schou, M. (1968) 'Lithium in psychiatric therapy and prophylaxis', *Journal of Psychiatric Research*, **6**, 67–69. This article was cited by *Current Contents* (September 1979) as a 'Citation Classic', i.e. an article cited by an exceptionally large number of authors since its publication.

78. Baastrup, personal communication (note 35).

79. Baastrup, personal communication (note 58).

80. Schou *et al.*, 'The treatment of manic psychoses by the administration of lithium salts' (note 12).
81. Trautner, E. M. (1954). Letter to M. Schou, 15 August.
82. Hartigan did not live to see the controversy which was provoked by his work. On 8 October 1968, Schou received a letter from Mrs Elizabeth Hartigan informing him of her husband's death some three months earlier. Schou immediately wrote to Mrs Hartigan with an elegant appreciation of her late husband and his work:

> It has indeed made me very, very sad to hear about your husband's sudden death. The death of a friend and colleague is always saddening, especially when he is of one's own age, but I consider this is a particularly severe loss for myself and for psychiatry. I am not familiar with your husband's other contributions, but his observation of the prophylactic lithium action against recurrent depressions unquestionably places him among the psychiatric pioneers. He and Dr Baastrup, simultaneously and quite independently of each other, saw something that was entirely unexpected and in a way highly unlikely, But as a true clinician your husband believed what his own eyes told him, and the more praise to him for that. His extreme modesty perhaps prevented him to some extent from getting all the general recognition he deserved, but I am particularly happy that he did publish that important paper in 1963. It may interest you to know that during the last four years it has been used in Danish Post Graduate Courses in Psychiatry as an illustration of the value of straightforward clinical observations, presented directly and without all statistical trimmings.
>
> Your husband's contribution will remain one of the milestones in psychiatry, and his observation has been instrumental in giving help to many, many patients who suffer from this terrible disorder. My own brother is among them, and I am truly grateful to your husband.
>
> I only met Dr Hartigan twice, in Chartham when I had the privilege of visiting your home, and on a later occasion in Birmingham. Even this brief acquaintance, combined, of course, with our correspondence, gave me a strong impression of his honesty, sincerity and sense of humour and human values. I mourn our loss and want to assure you of my sincere sympathy (Schou, M. (1968). Letter to Mrs E. Hartigan, 11 October.) See also note 38.

7 The therapeutic myth

1. Dr Blackwell left the Maudsley Hospital in 1968 and went to the USA where he is now a member of the Psychiatry Department at Mount Sinai Medical Center, Milwaukee, Wisconsin.
2. Blackwell, B. and Shepherd, M. (1968) 'Prophylactic lithium: another therapeutic myth? An examination of the evidence to date', *Lancet*, **i**, 968–71.
3. Baastrup, P. C. and Schou, M. (1967) 'Lithium as a prophylactic agent. Its effect against recurrent depressions and manic–depressive psychosis', *Archives of General Psychiatry*, **16**, 162–72.
4. Blackwell and Shepherd, 'Prophylactic lithium: another therapeutic myth?', 968 (note 2).
5. Ibid., 969. In the original passage a series of footnote references indicated which patients were being referred to, as identified by the code numbers used by Baastrup and Schou in their article 'Lithium as a prophylactic agent' (note 3).
6. Blackwell and Shepherd, 'Prophylactic lithium: another therapeutic myth?', 969 (note 2).

7. Ibid., 970.
8. Blackwell, B. (1980). Personal communication, 15 December.
9. Baastrup, P. C. and Schou, M. (1968) 'Prophylactic lithium', *Lancet*, **i**, 1419–22.
10. Ibid., 1420.
11. Ibid.
12. Ibid.
13. Hullin, R. P., McDonald, R., Anderson, W. McC. and Geraghty, S. M. J. (1968) 'Prophylactic lithium', *Lancet*, **i**, 1155–56.
14. Laurell, B. and Ottosson, J. O. (1968) 'Prophylactic lithium?', *Lancet*, **ii**, 1245–46.
15. Ibid., 1245.
16. Ibid.
17. Fieve, R. R. and Platman, S. R. (1968) 'Prophylactic lithium?', *Lancet*, **i**, 830.
18. Ibid.
19. Ibid.
20. Lader, M. H. (1968) 'Prophylactic lithium', *Lancet*, **ii**, 103.
21. Ibid.
22. Ibid.
23. See p. 76.
24. Baastrup, P. C. and Schou, M. (1968) 'Prophylactic lithium?' *Lancet*, **ii**, 349–50.
25. Sargant, W. (1968) 'Prophylactic lithium?' *Lancet*, **ii**, 216.
26. Kline, N. S. (1968) 'Lithium comes into its own', *American Journal of Psychiatry*, **125**, 558–60.
27. Ibid., 558.
28. Ibid.
29. Ibid., 559.
30. Blackwell, B. (1969) 'Need for careful evaluation of lithium', *American Journal of Psychiatry*, **125**, 1131.
31. Kline, N. S. (1969) 'Dr Kline replies', *American Journal of Psychiatry*, **125**, 1311.
32. Blackwell, B. (1969) 'Lithium: prophylactic or panacea?', *Medical Counterpoint*, November, 52–59.
33. Ibid., 52.
34. Ibid., 54.
35. Ibid., 56.
36. Ibid., 52.
37. Ibid., 59.
38. Shepherd, M. (1970–71) 'A prophylactic myth', *International Journal of Pychiatry*, **9**, 423–25.
39. Ibid., 425.
40. Shull, W. K. and Sapira, J. D. (1970) 'Critique of studies of lithium salts in the treatment of mania', *American Journal of Psychiatry*, **127**, 218–22.
41. Schou, M. (1982). Conversation, 18 April.
42. Ibid.
43. Ibid.
44. Ibid.
45. Schou, M. (1974) 'Ethical problems of therapeutic and prophylactic trials in manic–depressive disorder'. In, Bohaček, N. and Mihovilovič, M. (eds) *Psihofarmakologija 3: Proceedings of the 3rd Yugoslav Psychopharmocological Symposium, Opatija, 1973* (Zagreb: Medicinska Naklada) 323–28. Quotation from 325–26.
46. Ibid., 326.

47. Baastrup, P. C., Poulsen, J. C., Schou, M., Thomsen, K. and Amdisen, A. (1970) 'Prophylactic lithium: double-blind discontinuation in manic–depressive and recurrent–depressive disorders,' *Lancet*, **ii**, 326–30.
48. Schou, M. (1982). Personal communication, 20 December.
49. Blackwell, B. (1970) 'Lithium', *Lancet*, **ii**, 875.
50. Schou, M. (1970) 'Lithium', *Lancet*, **ii**, 875–76.
51. Mantel, N. (1971) 'Prophylactic lithium', *Lancet*, **i**, 758; Schou, M. and Thomsen, K. (1971) 'Prophylactic lithium', *Lancet*, **i**, 1066; Armitage, P. (1971) 'Prophylactic lithium', *Lancet*, **i**, 1066; Mantel, N. (1971) 'Sequential methods in clinical trials', *Lancet*, **i**, 1182–83.
52. Blackwell, B. (1972) 'Prophylactic lithium: science or science fiction?', *American Heart Journal*, **83**, 139–41.
53. Ibid., 140.
54. Blackwell, (1980). Personal communication, 15 December.
55. Shepherd, M. (1974) 'Discussion'. In, Bohaček and Mihovilovič, M. (eds) *Psihofarmakologija 3: Proceedings of the 3rd Yugoslav Psychopharmacological Symposium, Opatija, 1973* (Zagreb: Medicinska Noklada) 329–30. Quotation from 329.
56. Ibid., 330.
57. Baastrup and Schou, 'Prophylactic lithium' (note 9).
58. Blackwell and Shepherd, 'Prophylactic lithium: another therapeutic myth?' (note 2).
59. Schou, M. (1974) 'Discussion'. In, Bohaček, N. and Mihovilovič, M. (eds) *Psihofarmakologija 3: Proceedings of the 3rd Yugoslav Psychopharmacological Symposium, Opatija, 1973* (Zagreb: Medicinska Noklada) 330–32. Quotation from 331.
60. Anon (1969) 'Lithium', *Lancet*, **i**, 709–10.
61. The editor of the *Lancet* at the time was Dr Ian Douglas-Wilson. Professor W. Linford Rees recalls the events clearly.

   In 1970 Professor Schou told me that the *Lancet* had rejected his papers and I felt this was very unfortunate as they had published other papers which were detrimental to lithium therapy. When I got back to London from the conference in the Caribbean which Professor Schou and I attended, I spoke to the editor of the Lancet and he told me that he felt that lithium had received enough publicity. I firmly told him that it was very important because of its scientific value and because it was important that all the evidence regarding lithium should be made available to the medical profession. He then agreed to publish the paper. (Rees, W. L. (1982). Personal communication, 23 April).

62. Schou, M., Thomsen, K. and Baastrup, P. C. (1970) 'Studies on the course of recurrent endogenous affective disorders', *International Pharmacopsychiatry*, **5**, 100–06.
63. Schou, conversation (note 41).
64. The error appears in line 11 of the left-hand column on page 328 of Baastrup *et al.*, 'Prophylactic lithium: double-blind discontinuation in manic–depressive and recurrent–depressive disorders' (note 47).
65. Anon (1968) 'Lithium in psychiatric disorders', *British Medical Journal*, **4**, 271–72.
66. Anon (1970) 'Prophylactic lithium', *British Medical Journal*, **3**, 479–80.
67. Anon (1968) 'Lithium in mental disease', *British Medical Journal*, **4**, 502; Anon (1969) 'Lithium in mental disorders', *British Medical Journal*, **2**, 41.
68. Cade, J. F. J. (1970). Letter to M. Schou, 6 November.
69. Ibid.

70. *Psychological Medicine.*
71. Schou, M. and Strömgren, E. (eds) (1979) *Origin, Prevention and Treatment of Affective Disorders* (London: Academic Press).
72. Anon (1980) *Psychological Medicine*, May, 387.
73. Kline, N. S. (1982). Personal communication, 7 June.
74. Medical Research Council Drug Trials Subcommittee (1981) 'Continuation therapy with lithium and amitriptyline in unipolar depressive illness: a controlled trial', *Psychological Medicine*, **11**, 409–16.
75. The principles of prophylactic trials which had been so well worked out by Jules Angst and Paul Grof were subsequently presented in a form applicable to trials of all substances which have a suspected prophylactic effect: Grof, P., Schou, M., Angst, J., Baastrup, P. C. and Weis, P. (1970) 'Methodological problems of prophylactic trials in recurrent affective disorders', *British Journal of Psychiatry*, **116**, 599–619.
76. Schou, M. (1973) 'Prophylactic lithium maintenance treatment in recurrent endogenous affective disorders'. In, Gershon, S. and Shopsin, B. (eds) *Lithium: Its Role in Psychiatric Research and Treatment* (New York: Plenum) 269–94. Quotation from 286–87.
77. Schou, M. (1982). Personal communication, 20 December.

8 The spread of lithium therapy

1. Samuel Gershon, an Australian by birth, received his medical training at the University of Sydney and was a Resident in Psychiatry at various hospitals in Victoria. He became Professor of Psychiatry in the University of Melbourne, before moving to New York University Medical School in 1965. He is currently Professor and Chairman of Wayne State University School of Medicine, Department of Psychiatry, Detroit, as well as being Director of the Lafayette Clinic in the same city.
2. Gershon, S. and Yuwiler, A. (1960) 'A specific psychopharmacological approach to the treatment of mania', *Journal of Neuropsychiatry*, **1**, 229–41.
3. Robert F. Prien is a Research Psychologist in the Psychopharmacology Research Branch of the National Institute of Mental Health. In collaboration with E. M. Caffey and C. F. Klett he has directed the VA-NIMH collaborative study of lithium therapy which still represents the largest study on the clinical effectiveness of lithium.
4. Joyce G. Small is Professor of Psychiatry at the Indiana University School of Medicine, Larue D. Carter Memorial Hospital, Indianapolis.
5. Andrew K. S. Ho is particularly known for his work on lithium and alcohol preference.
6. Fieve, R. R. (1980). Personal communication, 9 December.
7. Kingstone, E. (1960) 'The lithium treatment of hypomanic and manic states', *Comprehensive Psychiatry*, **1**, 317–30. At the time of appearance of his article, Kingstone was a Travelling Fellow at the Institute of Psychiatry, Maudsley Hospital, London. In his article, the author wrote that 'to our knowledge, no report exists of lithium having been used in North America' (p. 317); this was true, although the general review written by Gershon and Yuwiler (see note 2) had been published whilst Kingstone's article was in press.
8. Fieve, R. P. (1975) *Moodswing: The Third Revolution in Psychiatry* (New York: William Morrow).
9. Fieve, personal communication (note 6).
10. Gershon, S. (1982). Personal communication, 23 December.
11. The forces which are at work to determine public acceptance of medical

treatments are frequently bizarre and unexpected. Dr. A. G. Awad (1980). Personal communication, 3 November, has given a nice example:

> There was an interesting, popular, and successful comedy series on North American television, called 'Maude' in which the main character was the erratic but charming Maude Finlay. This major character in the comedy was portrayed as suffering from manic–depressive illness and taking lithium. The show ran for several years and is now in reruns. I believe it has contributed to the acceptability of lithium therapy.

12. Schlagenhauf, C., Tupin, J. and White, R. B. (1966) 'The use of lithium carbonate in the treatment of manic psychoses', *American Journal of Psychiatry*, **123**, 201–06.
13. Warton, R. N. and Fieve, R. R. (1966) 'The use of lithium in the affective psychoses', *American Journal of Psychiatry*, **123**, 706–12.
14. Fieve, personal communication (note 6).
15. Joe P. Tupin, Professor of Psychiatry in the UCD Medical Center, Department of Psychiatry, Sacramento, California, is particularly known for his work on lithium and aggressiveness.
16. Tupin, J. P. (1980). Personal communication, 6 September.
17. Ibid.
18. Schlagenhauf *et al.*, 'The use of lithium carbonate in the treatment of manic psychoses' (note 12).
19. Goodman, L. S. and Gilman, A. (eds) (1956) *The Pharmacological Basis of Therapeutics* (New York: Macmillan).
20. Ibid., 817.
21. Wingard, C. (1961) 'Lithium salts', *Journal of the American Medical Association*, **175**, 340.
22. Prien, R. F. (1980). Personal communication, 6 October.
23. Gershon and Yuwiler, 'A specific psychopharmacological approach to the treatment of mania' (note 2)
24. Kingstone, 'The lithium treatment of hypomanic and manic states' (note 7).
25. At the time, Jonathon Cole was Director of the Psychopharmacology Service Center at the National Institute of Mental Health. Now Chief of the Psychopharmacology Program at McLean Hospital, Belmont, Massachusetts, Cole is modest about any influence which he might have had on the development of lithium therapy.

> I am not sure of my role in introducing lithium to the United States. I was certainly always positive about it, being brain-washed by Sam Gershon during his first tour in the United States in, I think, 1957–59 at Ypsilanti State Hospital and I believe NIMH supported individual studies before the large VA-NIMH collaborative study which was conceived before I left NIMH in 1967 but begun later (Cole, J. O. (1982). Personal communication, 14 June).

26. Cole, J. O. (1968) 'Lithium carbonate: some recommendations', *American Journal of Psychiatry*, **125**, 556–57.
27. Ibid., 556. In a personal communication (see note 25) Cole explains the background to this statement:

> The unsung hero of the introduction of lithium in the US was Dr Merle Gibson who was head of the FDA's Neuropharmacology Branch for (?) 5 years leading up to the eventual marketing of lithium carbonate by SKF, Pfizer and Rowell Labs. He decided to give individual IND numbers to a

very large number of psychiatrists interested in using lithium clinically and getting the drug dosages made in local drug stores or by Rowell Labs – they were, I think, the first company willing to make drug and placebo.

28. Cole, 'Lithium carbonate: some recommendations', 556–57 (note 26).
29. Ibid., 557.
30. Ibid.
31. Kline, N. S. (1981). Personal communication, 4 August.
32. Cole, 'Lithium carbonate: some recommendations', 557 (note 26).
33. FDA (1970) 'Lithium carbonate', *FDA Current Drug Information*, April.
34. Anon (1970) 'Current drug information', *Annals of Internal Medicine*, **73**, 291–93. Jonathon Cole has provided an intriguing background comment (personal communication, note 25):

> By the time that companies got approved NDAs and were able to sell lithium my guess is that most major cities in the US had one or more psychiatrists able to treat patients with lithium under an IND. [Dr Merle Gibson of the FDA] and I (I think) both encouraged companies to bite the fiscal bullet and market lithium. I was irked. Ben Greenwall at Rowell Labs, a small firm in upper Minnesota on a lake rich in fish with superior livers (for vitamin D) had forged ahead being helpful early to investigators. He believed Rowell was held up from releasing lithium for a year while SKF and Pfizer got their applications for NDAs in order.

35. FDA, 'Lithium carbonate' (note 33).
36. Ibid.
37. Prien, R. F., Klett, C. J. and Caffey, E. M. (1974) 'Lithium prophylaxis in recurrent affective illness', *American Journal of Psychiatry*, **131**, 192–96; Prien, R. F. and Caffey, E. M. (1976) 'Relationship between dosage and response to lithium prophylaxis in recurrent depression', *American Journal of Psychiatry*, **133**, 567–70.
38. Jonathon M. Himmelhoch is Professor of Psychiatry at the University of Pittsburgh School of Medicine.
39. Himmelhoch, J. M. (1980). Personal communication, 29 August.
40. Professor P. Stokes is at the Psychobiology Research Unit in Cornell University Medical College, Department of Psychiatry, New York.
41. Stokes, P. (1980). Personal communication, 8 September.
42. Tupin, personal communication (note 16).
43. Gershon, S. (1980). Personal communication, 10 November.
44. Prien, personal communication (note 22).
45. Himmelhoch, personal communication (note 39).
46. Rice, D. (1956) 'The use of lithium salts in the treatment of manic states', *Journal of Mental Science*, **102**, 604–11.
47. Rice, D. (1982). Personal communication, 19 April.
48. Dr Rice could not, unfortunately, recall the name of this interesting figure. The Australian connection seemed potentially important, however, and enquiries made to the Hospital Secretary at Graylingwell Hospital reached Dr Peter Sainsbury, Director of the MRC Clinical Psychiatry Unit based at the hospital. Dr Sainsbury said that two of the psychiatrists in the unit, Dr Morrissey and Dr Towers, remembered the Australian registrar as a Dr Moore, though no initials were recalled. Dr Moore apparently arrived in the hospital in or around 1949 armed with some papers on lithium therapy taken from the *Medical Journal of Australia* (presumably the articles of Cade or Trautner). When the Royal Australian and New Zealand College of Psychiatrists were contacted to see whether a Dr Moore was listed amongst the college's membership, only one likely candidate emerged, but the trail proved to be a false one.

A third line of enquiry was to the editor of the *Australian and New Zealand Journal of Medicine* who passed on the query to Professor H. D. Attwood, Curator of the Medical History Unit in the University of Melbourne. This time the response was positive. Professor Attwood wrote, 'I believe that the Dr Moore you have been seeking was David Robert Moore who died in Longford, Tasmania, in 1979. He moved to Tasmania in 1975 having worked as a psychiatrist at the Ernest Jones Clinic, 85 Hotham Street, Preston, Victoria 3072, Australia' (Attwood, H. D. (1982). Personal communication, 9 July).

49. Actually, it must have been the *Medical Journal of Australia*.
50. In his published article 'The use of lithium salts in the treatment of manic states' (note 46), Rice had said that it was the Noack and Trautner article which had been produced:

My attention was drawn in 1952 to the paper by Noack and Trautner which had appeared the previous year, reporting the use of lithium in the treatment of maniacal psychosis and since their findings appeared to substantiate other claims, notably those of Cade and Ashburner, it was resolved to try the use of lithium in a few manic patients who for one reason of another presented especial difficulty' (p. 605).

51. Maggs, R. (1982). Personal communication, 18 April. David Rice, however, notes that Dr Moore did not actually describe anything; he merely showed Rice the article. Moore was, as Rice recalls 'a pretty retiring, silent chap' (Rice, D. (1982). Personal communication, 23 December).
52. Rice, (1982). Personal communication, 19 April. Though in a later personal communication (23 December 1982) Rice notes that he had just taken over as Medical Superintendent and it was the large administrative load which he carried that really stopped him getting involved with Maggs' study. 'I couldn't have *planned* a trial', said Rice 'but without the load I could have joined in Ronnie's work.'
53. Maggs, R. (1963) 'Treatment of manic illness with lithium carbonate', *British Journal of Psychiatry*, **109**, 56–65.
54. Rice, (1982). Personal communication 23 December: 'I knew Hartigan who told me it was my article which stimulated his interest.'
55. This was the first time that Maggs and Schou had met, though they had corresponded on a number of occasions.
56. Maggs, personal communication (note 51).
57. Hellingly, Epsom, Surrey; Bethlem Royal and Maudsley Hospitals, Beckenham, Kent; and Hollymoor Hospital, Northfield, Birmingham: Coppen, A., Noguera, R., Bailey, J., Burns, B. H., Swami, M. S., Mare, E. H., Gardner, R. and Maggs, R. (1971) 'Prophylactic lithium in affective disorders' *Lancet*, **ii**, 275–79.
58. Blackwell, B. and Shepherd, M. (1968) 'Prophylactic lithium: another therapeutic myth? An examination of the evidence to date', *Lancet*, **i**, 968–71.
59. See p. 96
60. Kingstone, 'The lithium treatment of hypomanic and manic states' (note 7).
61. Dr D. Ewen Cameron introduced the idea of treating senile dementia and arteriosclerotic dementia with RNA.
62. Kingstone, E. (1976) 'The history and current status of lithium in Canada'. In, Villeneuve, A. (ed.) *Lithium in Psychiatry: A Synopsis*. Proceedings of the First Canadian International Symposium on Lithium, Quebec 24 May 1974 (Quebec: Les Presses de l'Université Laval) 79–92; this extract, 81–82.
63. Ibid., 82–83.
64. Ibid., 83.
65. Ibid., 83–84.

66. See pp. 39–41.
67. Kingstone, 'The history and current status of lithium in Canada', 84 (note 62).
68. Hartigan, G. P. (1963) 'The use of lithium salts in affective disorders', *British Journal of Psychiatry*, **109**, 810–14.
69. Melia, P. I. (1967) 'A pilot trial of lithium carbonate in recurrent affective disorders', *Journal of the Irish Medical Association*, **40**, 160–70.
70. Melia, P. I. (1968) 'Prophylactic lithium', *Lancet*, **ii**, 519–20.
71. Melia, P. I. (1970) 'Prophylactic lithium – a double-blind trial in recurrent affective disorders', *British Journal of Psychiatry*, **116**, 621–24.
72. Christodolou, G. N. (1967) 'Applications of lithium in psychiatry', [in Greek] *Iatriki*, **11**, 486–93. This was the first article on the psychiatric uses of lithium to be published in Greece. Christodolou, G. N. (1968) 'Lithium in clinical practice', [in Greek] *Acta Neurologica et Psychiatrica Hellenica*, **7**, 122–33. This was the first publication in Greece to deal with original observations (on both acute and prophylactic uses of lithium).
73. Professor Lopez-Ibor Aliño opened the first lithium clinic in Spain in 1969. In 1970 he published a long review which brought lithium therapy to the attention of Spanish psychiatrists and which must certainly have been widely read in the Spanish-speaking countries of Latin America: Lopez-Ibor Aliño, J. J. (1970) 'Empleo del litio en los trastornos mentales: situacion actual y experimental propia', *Actas Luso-Espanolas de Neurologia y Psiquiatria*, **24**, 197–242.
74. Dr Athanasio Kukopulos heads a talented and productive team of psychiatrists working mainly in Rome and Cagliari, Sardinia.
75. Kukopulos, A. (1981). Personal communication, 3 February.
76. Gershon, E. S. (1980). Personal communication, 4 August.
77. Cade, J. F. J. (1949) 'Lithium salts in the treatment of psychotic excitement', *Medical Journal of Australia*, **36**, 349–52.
78. Hanzliček, L. (1957) 'Lithiove soli v psychiatrii'. In, *Problemy Psychiatrie v Praxi a ve Vyzkumu* (Prague: Czechoslovak Medical Press) 60–61. Dr Hanzliček is now Director of the Psychiatric Research Institute in Prague.
79. Grof, P. (1983). Personal communication, 21 January.
80. Zvolsky, P. (1981). Personal communication, 18 April.
81. Drs Jaromio Svestka, Karel Nahunek and A. Radova, in particular, are very active in lithium research. Their first publication was in 1970: Svestka, J., Nahunek, K. and Radova, A. (1970) 'Side effects and complications in lithium therapy', *Activitas Nervosa Superior*, **12**, 264–65; though their interest in lithium as an antimanic treatment predated this by some years.
82. Yan Shanming (1981) 'Lithium therapy in China', *Acta Psychiatrica Scandinavica*, **64**, 270–72.
83. Yan Shanming (1982). Personal communication, 28 March.
84. Yan Shanming, 'Lithium therapy in China' (note 82).
85. Yan Shanming, personal communication (note 83).

9 Developments and crises

1. Cade, J. F. J. (1970) 'The story of lithium'. In, Ayd, F. J. (ed.) *Discoveries in Biological Psychiatry* (Philadelphia: Lippincott) 218–29. Quotation from 220.
2. Cade, J. F. J. (1949) 'Lithium salts in the treatment of manic excitement', *Medical Journal of Australia*, **36**, 349–52.
3. Noack, C. H. and Trautner, E. M. (1951) 'The lithium treatment of maniacal psychoses', *Medical Journal of Australia*, **38**, 219–22.
4. Ibid.

5. Schou, M. (1959) 'Lithium in psychiatric therapy: stock-taking after ten years', *Psychopharmacologia*, **1**, 65–78.
6. The unpublished study was credited to C. J. Hansen, K. Retbøll and M. Schou.
7. Schou, 'Lithium in psychiatric therapy', 72 (note 5).
8. Ibid.
9. Vojtechovsky, M. (1957) 'Zkusenosti s lecbou solemi lithia.' In, *Problemy Psychiatrie v Praxi a ve Vyzkumu* (Prague: Czechoslovak Medical Press) pp. 216–24.
10. Andreani, G., Caselli, G. and Martelli, G. (1958) 'Rilievi clinici ed elettroence-falografici durante il trattamento con sali de litio in malati psichiatric', *Giornal di Psichiatria e Neuropathologica*, **86**, 273–328.
11. Fieve, R. R., Platman, S. R. and Plutchik, R. R. (1968) 'The use of lithium in affective disorders: I. Acute endogenous depression', *American Journal of Psychiatry*, **125**, 487–91.
12. Ibid., 491.
13. Schou, M. (1968) 'Lithium in psychiatric therapy and prophylaxis', *Journal of Psychiatric Research*, **6**, 67–95. Quotation from 76.
14. Dyson, W. L. and Mendelson, M. (1968) 'Recurrent depressions and the lithium ion', *American Journal of Psychiatry*, **125**, 544–49.
15. Ibid., 544.
16. Dyson, W. L. and Mendels, J. (1968) 'Lithium and depression', *Current Therapeutic Research*, **10**, 601–08.
17. Goodwin, F. K., Murphy, D. L. and Bunney, W. E. Jr (1969) 'Lithium', *Lancet*, **ii**, 212–13.
18. Ibid., 213.
19. Ibid.
20. Van der Velde, C. D. (1970) 'Effectiveness of lithium carbonate in the treatment of manic–depressive illness', *American Journal of Psychiatry*, **127**, 345–51; Stokes, P. E., Stoll, P. M., Shamoian, C. A. and Patton, M. J. (1971) 'Efficacy of lithium as an acute treatment of manic–depressive illness', *Lancet*, **i**, 1319–25.
21. Mendels, J., Secunda, S. K. and Dyson, W. L. (1972) 'A controlled study of the antidepressant effects of lithium carbonate', *Archives of General Psychiatry*, **26**, 154–57.
22. For example: Baron, M., Gershon, E. S., Rudy, V., Jonas, W. Z. and Buchsbaum, M. (1975) 'Lithium carbonate response in depression: prediction by unipolar/bipolar illness, average-evoked response, catechol-O-methyl transferase, and family history', *Archives of General Psychiatry*, **32**, 1107–11.
23. Peet, M. and Coppen, A. (1980) 'Lithium treatment and prophylaxis in unipolar depression', *Psychosomatics*, **21**, 303–13. Quotation from 309.
24. Mendels, J. (1982). Personal communication, 21 December.
25. Ibid.
26. Ibid.
27. See pp. 60–64.
28. Lange, F. (1894) *De vigtigste Sindssygdomsgrupper.* (Copenhagen: Gyldendalske Boghandels Forlag).
29. Cade, 'The story of lithium' (note 1).
30. Watanabe, S. and Ishino, H. (1980) 'Special cases of affective disorder and their treatment with lithium'. In, Johnson, F. N. (ed.) *Handbook of Lithium Therapy* (Lancaster: MTP Press) 39–46. Quotation from 43.
31. Cade, 'The story of lithium' (note 1).
32. Annell, A-L. (1969) 'Lithium in the treatment of children and adolescents', *Acta Psychiatria Scandinavica*, Suppl. 207, 19–33; Forssman, H. and Wålin-

der, J. (1969) 'Lithium treatment on a typical indication', *Acta Psychiatria Scandinavica*, Suppl. 207, 34–40.

33. Dostal, T. and Zvolsky, P. (1970) 'Anti-aggressive effect of lithium salts in severe mentally retarded adolescents', *International Pharmacopsychiatry*, **5**, 203–07.

34. Sheard, M. H. (1971) 'Effect of lithium on human aggression', *Nature*, **230**, 113–14. Dr Joe Tupin has also been particularly involved in this area: Tupin, J. P. and Smith, D. B. (1973) 'The long-term use of lithium in aggressive prisoners', *Psychopharmacology Bulletin*, **9**, 48; Tupin, J. P., Smith, D. B., Clanon, T. L., Kim, L. I., Nugent, A. and Groupe, A. (1973) 'The long-term use of lithium in aggressive prisoners', *Comprehensive Psychiatry*, **14**, 311–17.

35. Wren, J. C., Kline, N. S., Cooper, T. B., Varga, E. and Canal, O. (1974) 'Evaluation of lithium therapy in chronic alcoholism', *Clinical Medicine*, **81**, 33–361; Kline, N. S., Wren, J. C., Cooper, T. B., Varga, E. and Canal, O. (1974) 'Evaluation of lithium therapy in chronic and periodic alcoholism', *American Journal of the Medical Sciences*, **268**, 15–22; Kline, N. S. and Cooper, T. B. (1974) 'Lithium as a possible therapeutic agent in the treatment of chronic periodic alcoholism', *Interface*, **3**, 16.

36. Wren *et al.* 'Evaluation of lithium therapy in chronic alcoholism', 33 (note 35).

37. Kline *et al.* 'Evaluation of lithium therapy in chronic and periodic alcoholism', 21 (note 35).

38. Fries, H. (1969) 'Experience with lithium carbonate treatment at a psychiatric department in the period 1964–67', *Acta Psychiatrica Scandinavia*, **207**, 41–43.

39. Ibid., 42.

40. Kline *et al.* 'Evaluation of lithium therapy in chronic and periodic alcoholism', 21 (note 35).

41. Sinclair, J. D. (1974) 'Lithium-induced suppression of alcohol drinking by rats', *Medical Biology*, **52**, 133–36.

42. Sinclair, J. D. (1980). Personal communication, 23 November.

43. Ho, A. K. S. (1980). Personal communication, 3 October; Ho, A. K. S. and Tsai, C. S. (1975) 'Lithium and alcohol preference', *Journal of Pharmacy and Pharmacology*, **27**, 58–59.

44. Reynolds, C. M., Merry, J. and Coppen, A. (1977) 'Prophylactic treatment of alcoholism by lithium carbonate: an initial report'. *Alcoholism: Clinical and Experimental Research*, **1**, 109–11.

45. Ho, personal communication (note 43).

46. Sinclair, personal communication (note 42).

47. Ibid.

48. Schou, M. (1980) 'The range of non-psychiatric uses of lithium'. In, Johnson, F. N. (ed.) *Handbook of Lithium Therapy* (Lancaster: MTP Press) 73–79.

49. Johnson, F. N. (1980) 'The choice of an appropriate lithium preparation'. In, Johnson, F. N. (ed.) *Handbook of Lithium Therapy* (Lancaster: MTP Press) 225–36.

50. Amdisen, A. (1980). Personal communication, 18 August.

51. Ibid.

52. See p. 17.

53. Cooper, T. B. (1980) 'Monitoring lithium dose levels: estimation of lithium in blood'. In, Johnson, F. N. (ed.) *Handbook of Lithium Therapy* (Lancaster: MTP Press) 169–78.

54. Amdisen, A. (1980) 'Monitoring lithium dose levels: estimation of lithium in urine'. In, Johnson, F. N. (ed.) *Handbook of Lithium Therapy* (Lancaster: MTP Press) 196–99.

55. Sims, A. (1980) 'Monitoring lithium dose levels: estimation of lithium in saliva'. In, Johnson, F. N. (ed.) *Handbook of Lithium Therapy* (Lancaster: MTP Press) 200–04.
56. See pp. 46–57.
57. Sedvall, G., Jonsson, B. and Pettersson, U. (1969) 'Evidence of an altered thyroid function in man during treatment with lithium carbonate', *Acta Psychiatrica Scandinavica*, Suppl. 207, 59–67. Quotation from 59.
58. Amdisen, personal communication (note 50).
59. Schou, 'Lithium in psychiatric therapy and prophylaxis' (note 13).
60. Amdisen, A. Eskjaer-Jensen, S., Olsen, T. and Schou, M. (1968) 'Forekomst af struma under lithiumbehandling', *Ugeskrift for Laeger*, **130**, 1515–18.
61. In addition to the clinical report (Amdisen *et al.* 'Forekomst of struma under lithiumbehandling', note 60) Amdisen, in association with others, published data on iodine metabolism under lithium therapy: Eskjaer-Jensen, S., Amdisen, A., Olsen, T. and Schou, M. (1968) 'Jodstofskiftet under lithiumbehandling', *Ugeskrift for Laeger*, **130**, 1518–20.

    A symposium on lithium and goitre had been held at Aarhus University, Risskov, in Denmark, in 1967; at this symposium there were reports of patients on long-term lithium treatment who had developed diffuse thyroid enlargements (Allgen, L.-G., Almgren, S. and Martens, S. (1967). Unpublished communication. Symposium on Lithium and Goitre, Risskov, Denmark; Baastrup, P. C. (1967). Unpublished communication. Symposium on Lithium and Goitre, Risskov, Denmark).
62. Sedvall, G., Jonsson, B., Pettersson, U. and Levin, K. (1968) 'Effects of lithium salts on plasma protein-bound iodine and uptake of I^{131} in thyroid gland of man and rat', *Life Sciences*, **7**, 1257–64.
63. Männistö, P. T. (1980) 'Endocrine side-effects of lithium'. In, Johnson, F. N. (ed.) *Handbook of Lithium Therapy* (Lancaster: MTP Press) 310–22.
64. Weinstein, M. R. and Goldfield, M. (1969) 'Lithium carbonate treatment during pregnancy. Report of a case', *Diseases of the Nervous System*, **30**, 833–42.
65. Schou had stated briefly in 1968 (Schou, M. (1968) 'Lithium in psychiatry – a review'. In, Efron, D. H., Cole, J. O., Levine, J. and Wittenborn, J. R. (eds) *Psychopharmacology. A Review of Progress 1957–1967*, PHS Publication No. 1836 (Washington: US Government Printing Office) 701–18) that he was aware of six normal babies conceived and born to mothers under continuous medication with lithium.
66. Weinstein and Goldfield 'Lithium carbonate treatment during pregnancy', 835–36 (note 64).
67. Weinstein, M. R. (1976) 'The international register of lithium babies', *Drug Information Journal*, **10**, 96–100.
68. At the present time the Register remains more or less inactive, though there are suggestions that it may be continued (Lannon, R. A. (1981). Personal communication, 7 January). However, Mogens Schou has indicated (Schou, M. (1980). Personal communication, 23 September) that this may not necessarily be a good thing.

Another question is whether it is in fact worth while to continue the Register. There are of course arguments in favour on this, but I feel that there are other arguments against. If the existence of the Register and the obligation of doctors to report to it are not constantly kept in people's minds, then there is a still larger risk that only abnormal cases are being reported and that the normal children are not. This will give still more bias than that already inherent in the retrospective procedure for collecting the data. I am therefore in considerable doubt whether the Register should be continued.

69. Weinstein, M. R. (1980) 'Lithium treatment of women during pregnancy and in the post-delivery period'. In, Johnson, F. N. (ed.) *Handbook of Lithium Therapy* (Lancaster: MTP Press) 421–29.
70. Schou, personal communication (note 68).
71. Weinstein, M. R. and Goldfield, M. D. (1975) 'Administration of lithium during pregnancy'. In, Johnson, F. N. (ed.) *Lithium Research and Therapy* (London: Academic Press) 237–64.
72. As early as 1863, A. B. Garrod had recorded the occurrence of polyuria and polydipsia during lithium administration in man. Garrod, A. B. (1863) *The Nature and Treatment of Gout and Rheumatic Gout*, 2nd edn (London: Walton and Maberly).
73. Amdisen, personal communication (note 50).
74. Schou, M. and Vestergaard, P. (1981) 'Lithium and the kidney scare', *Psychosomatics*, **22**, 92–94.
75. Hestbech, J., Hansen, H. E., Amdisen, A. and Olesen, S. (1977) 'Chronic renal lesions following long-term treatment with lithium', *Kidney International*, **12**, 205–13; Hansen, H. E., Hestbech, J., Olesen, S. and Amdisen, A. (1977) 'Renal function and renal pathology in patients with lithium-induced impairment of renal concentrating ability', *Proceedings of the European Dialysis and Transplantation Association*, **14**, 518–27.
76. Schou and Vestergaard, 'Lithium and the kidney scare', 92 (note 74).
77. Ibid.
78. Viol, G. W., Grof, P. and Daigle, L. (1975) 'Renal tubular function in patients on long-term lithium therapy', *American Journal of Psychiatry*, **132**, 68–69.
79. Kincaid-Smith, P., Burrows, G. D., Davies, B. M., Holwill, B., Walter, M. and Walker, R. E. (1979) 'Renal-biopsy findings in lithium and pre-lithium patients', *Lancet*, **ii**, 700–01.
80. Jenner, F. A. (1979) 'Lithium and the kidney'. In, Cooper, T. B., Gershon, S., Kline, N. S. and Schou, M. (eds) *Lithium: Controversies and Unresolved Issues* (Amsterdam: Excerpta Medica) 567–77. Quotation from 567.
81. Schou and Vestergaard, 'Lithium and the kidney scare', 94 (note 74).
82. Hansen, H. E. (1981) 'Renal toxicity of lithium', *Drugs*, **22**, 461–76. Quotation from 461–2.
83. Amdisen, A. (1982). Personal communication, 28 December.
84. Ibid.
85. Shopsin, B. (1978). Paper read at the International Lithium Conference, New York City, New York, 5–9 June. Subsequently reported in: Shopsin, B., Temple, H., Ingiver, M., Kane, S. and Hirsch, J. (1979) 'Sudden death during lithium carbonate maintenance'. In, Cooper, T. B., Gershon, S., Kline, N. S. and Schou, M. (eds) *Lithium: Controversies and Unresolved Issues* (Amsterdam: Excerpta Medica) 527–51.
86. See pp. 46–57.

10 The future

1. In 1967, Mogens Schou reported:

   In pharmacological tests lithium is strikingly different from the other psychotropic drugs. Studying the activity of mice we have not been able to note any effect of lithium administration even in very high doses. . . . Also in most of the other screening and characterisation of neuroleptics, tranquillisers, stimulants and antidepressives, lithium fails to show an effect when given in doses comparable to those used in psychiatric therapy. (Schou, M. (1967) 'Lithium, sodium and manic–depressive psychosis'. In, Waalaas, O. (ed.) *Molecular Basis of Some Aspects of Mental Activity*, Vol. 2 (London: Academic Press) 457–63. Quotation from 461).

Schou drew his evidence for these assertions from unpublished observations obtained in 1963 by himself and Amdi Amdisen, and from personal communications which he had received in the same year from D. R. Maxwell and I. Møller-Neilsen.

2. In 1963, Schou noted that the normothymotics (lithium and imipramine) 'do not influence the normal mind and do not level out normal emotions' (Schou, M. (1963) 'Normothymotics, "mood normalizers"', *British Journal of Psychiatry*, **109**, 803–09. Quotation from 808). Later, in 1968, writing with Drs Amdi Amdisen and Klaus Thomsen, Schou expanded this comment.

Even when given continuously for years this lithium dosage [25 mg per day] does not affect the normal mental functions. Neither consciousness nor memory are impaired, and intellectual productivity is unchanged. The emotional range is not restricted; patients in lithium treatment are able to feel happiness and sorrow to an entirely normal extent. (Schou, M., Amdisen, A. and Thomsen, K. (1968) 'The effect of lithium on the normal human mind'. In, Baudis, P., Peterova, E. and Sediveč, V. (eds) *De Psychiatria Progrediente*, Vol. 2 (Plzen.) 712–21. Quotation from 712).

3. See pp. 34–45.
4. Johnson, F. N. and Wormington, S. (1972) 'Effect of lithium on rearing activity in rats', *Nature New Biology*, **235**, 159–60.
5. Johnson, F. N. (1972) 'Dissociation of vertical and horizontal components of activity in rats treated with lithium chloride', *Experientia*, **28**, 533–35.
6. Johnson, F. N. (1972) 'Chlorpromazine and lithium: effects on stimulus significance', *Diseases of the Nervous System*, **33**, 235–41.
7. Johnson, F. N. (1975) 'Depression: some proposals for future research', *Disease of the Nervous System*, **36**, 228–32.
8. Referring to observations which they had made on the effects of lithium on the performance of normal volunteers on a variety of cognitive/motor performance tests, Lewis Judd and his colleagues at the University of California, San Diego, commented:

It is our feeling that the locus of lithium carbonate's effect in impairing performance is an important issue. Is it due to simple motor slowing or is it an effect that has more to do with a slowing in thinking or information processing? If the latter were true it would reveal something hitherto unnoticed about the overall effects of lithium carbonate. (Judd, L. L., Hubbard, B., Janowsky, D. S., Huey, L. Y. and Takahashi, K. I. (1977) 'The effect of lithium carbonate on the cognitive functions of normal subjects', *Archives of General Psychiatry*, **34**, 355–57.

Later work generally confirmed this view: the results obtained were taken to indicate that 'lithium exerts a central effect by slowing the rate of cognitive processing' and that 'this slowing of central cognitive processing could be one of the behavioural mechanisms by which lithium exerts a therapeutic effect during manic and hypomanic states' (Judd, L. L. (1979) 'Effect of lithium on mood, cognition, and personality function in normal subjects', *Archives of General Psychiatry*, **36**, 860–65. Quotations from 864).

The most recent evidence from humans which accords with the animal work was reported in Lund, Y., Nissen, M. and Rafaelsen, O. J. (1982) 'Long-term lithium treatment and psychological functions', *Acta Psychiatrica Scandinavica*, **65**, 233–44. These authors concluded that their study 'supports the evidence of a specific lithium-related effect on information processing' (p. 240).

9. Johnson, F. N. (1979) 'Animal behaviour studies involving lithium'. In, Cooper, T. B., Gershon, S., Kline, N. S. and Schou, M. (eds) *Lithium: Controversies and Unresolved Issues. Proceedings of the International Lithium Conference, New York, June 5–9, 1978.* (Amsterdam: Excerpta Medica) 945–95.

10. Ibid., 950.

Appendix

Experiences of treatment with lithium salts

G. P. Hartigan,
St Augustine's Hospital,
Chartham, Canterbury

The following is the full text of the paper read by Dr Hartigan to the Southeastern Branch of the Royal Medicopsychological Society in 1959, and never before published.

Although my acquaintance with lithium treatment is limited to relatively few cases (twenty in all) over a fairly short period of time, I have thought it worthwhile to bring to your notice my experiences with this drug. I believe that lithium has a specific place in psychiatric therapy and it is possible that its usefulness may prove to be even more extensive than is at present realised. Such is my excuse for recounting at this stage some scrappy and incomplete clinical data in the hope of stimulating interest in a potent, inexpensive and relatively safe drug.

A brief outline of the history and literature of the drug may be helpful. Apart from a slight and unimportant part in the treatment of gout and epilepsy lithium had never been found to be of any great therapeutic account. In the late 1940s however, it began to be used in a salt substitute in cardiac patients on a low-sodium diet. These unfortunates condemned to an unpalatable regimen were invited to sprinkle their food liberally with lithium salts. In some cases this resulted in ingestion of large doses of lithium and there were many serious complications, some of them fatal. The salt substitute was hastily withdrawn and lithium retired in deep disgrace into its previous obscurity. Shortly afterwards, however, it re-emerged in a very different setting. Some Australian physiologists, working on some recondite project whose exact nature I regret I am unable to recall, found it expedient to introduce a lithium salt into the peritoneal cavities of guinea-pigs. It was observed that for some hours after this outrage the animals became thoughtful and preoccupied. This really seems hardly surprising, but the phenomenon prompted the Australian psychiatrist Cade to use the substance therapeutically in a small group of excited psychotics. The results were unexpectedly gratifying, and from that time on considerable use was made of lithium salts in Australian psychiatry and a number of most useful papers, recording results in some hundreds of cases, was published. It seems that the treatment became widely adopted in Antipodean mental hospitals and is still much used as far as I can gather, although nothing from that quarter has been published since 1955. Other countries followed suit at a discreet distance. Those therapeutic jackals, the French, reported on its use in small groups of cases, but they were seduced from it by the arrival of their own more dramatic and far more expensive tranquilliser chlor-promazine. Lately the Italians have shown themselves interested, and there was a very good paper from Adreani da Ferrara in 1958. The Danish psychiatrist Schou of Aarhus has written a number of papers which provide the most convincing controlled material in the whole literature. The only writer on the use of the drug in this country is Rice of Hellingly, to whose stimulating article in the JMS of 1956 I owe my first introduction to lithium. There is stony silence on the topic from the other side of the Atlantic.

In all the literature to date there is recorded the treatment of over 1000 patients. With rare exceptions all authors are agreed that the drug has a specific effect on manic and hypnomanic [sic] states and in their prevention of relapses in recurrent cases. The results in other states of excitement, for instance, schizophrenia, epilepsy and oligophrenia, are equivocal, and other drugs or physical forms of treatment are probably at least as effective. The results obtained by most workers in depressive syndromes have not been encouraging, but I shall have something to say about that later on.

The significance of these findings may now be examined. Cases of acute manic excitement usually respond in time to various other forms of treatment, such as the organic tranquillisers or electrotherapy, and, as lithium is not a particularly rapidly acting drug, its usefulness in this state, although undoubted, is not especially dramatic. In cases of sustained hypnomania [sic] however, or even more remarkably in those cases in which frequent attacks of mania or hypomania recur with brief remissions, the drug has a specific effect. We are all familiar with the relapsing manic patient whose management is so difficult from the therapeutic, sociological and legal standpoints. A high percentage of these patients can be brought back to a normal affective state and maintained in it over long periods by lithium. In this relatively small field I believe that lithium is unequalled by any other drug or method of treatment at present in use.

The drug is usually given by mouth before meals in the form either of the carbonate (1–2 g daily in divided doses) or of the citrate (2–3 g daily). A few workers have given the citrate parenterally in 10 per cent solution. Dosage of this order usually starts to take effect in three or four days and may be expected to eliminate excitement rapidly in the next few days. A smaller dose is then used for maintenance; it is likely that the lowest effective dose for this purpose is 0.3 g of the carbonate b.d. If this is not done there is a strong possibility of relapse, and I have kept several patients on the drug for as long as two years and intend to continue the maintenance dose indefinitely. Toxic effects in the early stages are not uncommon. The first to appear are those of gastro-intestinal upset – anorexia, vomiting and diarrhoea, which usually pass off in a few days. Neurological symptoms may appear after about a week. The most common is a marked tremor of the hands; this usually subsides in a few weeks, especially if the dose can be reduced. Graver neurological symptoms, which are rare, take the form of various extra-pyramidal syndromes and may proceed by stupor into coma and death. In over 1000 cases of treatment described in the literature a total of nine deaths has been recorded. In two of these, renal function was known to be seriously deficient, and in one other the cause of death (pontine infarction) may have been incidental. Provided that renal and cardiac function are reasonably good and that an adequate sodium intake is maintained, the therapeutic dosage is sufficiently lower than the toxic one for the drug to be prescribed without anxiety to in-patients.

Smaller maintenance doses seem in my experience to be quite safe for out-patients over long periods. I have not myself encountered serious toxic symptoms, but it seems from the literature that a very few individuals are abnormally sensitive to the drug, and consequently it is best to initiate treatment in hospital whenever possible. I have not found estimations of serum lithium necessary in my cases, and, from the experience of other authors, they seem to have little protective value except in that very small number of patients who tend to retain lithium in the body to an abnormal extent.

In relating my own experiences with the drug I have decided to describe in brief the case histories of certain individual patients. I have not concerned myself with the problem of proving or disproving the efficacy of the drug from a scientific standpoint, as the numbers I have treated personally (only twenty) are insufficient for that purpose, and in any event, as I have indicated, several large-scale trials, some even with acceptable controls, have already been carried out by others. The long-term prognosis of recurrent affective disorders has been my principal interest, and it is far too early for me to assemble a sufficient number of cases treated and followed up for the necessary period of years which would enable me to ascribe with certainty curative and preventive properties to the treatment. I hope, however, that this anecdotal approach, though rightly much out of favour in academic circles, may be tolerated in as much as it may serve to indicate the types of patients who may be submitted to lithium therapy with a good prospect of a successful result.

The cases I have treated fall into three main diagnostic categories. Firstly there are cases of mania and hypomania, either sustained or remittent; these patients resemble closely those described in the literature as responding particularly well to lithium. Secondly there is a small group of cases exhibiting an extreme form of manic–depressive personality but falling short of the psychotic level at extremes. Thirdly I have treated by this method a number of cases of repeatedly recurring endogenous depression.

From the first group I have selected two examples. A man, then aged forty-five, was admitted to this hospital under certificate in May 1955 in a state of mania. He had had an unhappy childhood, his father being a drunkard and his mother embittered in consequence, but there was no family history of psychosis. At the age of seventeen, while at a Technical College, he had a severe manic attack and was admitted to another mental hospital under certificate. He recovered under treatment and subsequently took a BSc and MSc and obtained a post at a nearby agricultural institution. During the nearly thirty years which intervened between his first illness and his admission here in 1955 he had had two depressive episodes which had not come to medical notice. These were short-lived but severe, and during one of them he went to an orchard and put the muzzle of a shot-gun in his mouth, but happily for my series he did not press the trigger. On his first admission here in May 1955 his condition was that of a typical mania. He recovered completely with electroplexy and was discharged in September, but in November of the same year he had to be re-admitted, this time with a severe depression, which also responded to electroplexy. A month later there was an episode of hypomania necessitating his admission to hospital again. Here electroplexy, this time accompanied by chlorpromazine restored him to normal, but in August 1956 he had to have a nephrectomy and during convalescence became hypomanic again. Management of this phase was difficult, as he was far from cooperative, and he had to be in hospital for three months and to undergo many electrical treatments before he could again be discharged. A few weeks later, in November 1956 he had to be admitted again in a state of hypomania. He had four ECT and recovered his stability. By this time his wife was at her wits' end and his employers, who had been extremely tolerant, were not going to be able to stand much more. It was clear that electroplexy and chlorpromazine, although effective in ending an attack, were powerless to prevent the frequent recurrences which were having such serious social repercussions. After recovery from this latest attack I put him on lithium carbonate 0.6 t.d.s. [sic] – the first patient I had so treated. Chlorpromazine was discontinued. Since that day, now twenty-seven months ago, he has had no further episodes and is living a normal domestic and social life. The dose of lithium has been gradually reduced to 0.3 g b.d. which he is still taking.

This was a very gratifying outcome for one's first experience with a new drug. I have since treated nine similar cases with manic or hypomanic disorders, with completely satisfactory results in seven. A somewhat different type of case in the same group may be of interest to you. A woman of sixty-five was admitted to hospital in May of this year. Her parents had separated when she was fifteen, but there was no history of psychosis in the family. She was a well-educated woman and led a useful and interesting life. Her first husband died and she married again at the age of forty-two. When she was fifty-four her son got married and this event precipitated a long episode of overactivity, irritability and aggressiveness. There was some improvement after a time but she gradually passed into a chronic state of hypomania. She was interfering, vindictive, tactless, overbearing, inconsiderate, and altogether quite intolerable. She was extremely overactive, heedless of time, and she slept very little. Her husband, a long-suffering ex-hospital administrator who had been devoted to her, was on the brink of leaving her and she had alienated all her relatives and friends. At this time she was admitted to a general hospital with an obscure diarrhoea labelled 'colitis'. As her behaviour in the ward was so odd, I was asked to see her and managed to inviegle her into this hospital for the purpose of convalescence. She was at once put on lithium carbonate 0.3 g t.d.s. Her first few days in hospital were very trying. She was demanding, attention-seeking, restless, and aggressive. She had furious rows with the other patients. Within a month she had completely calmed down into a tranquil and even rather apathetic state. On discharge she continued in her reposeful mood and began to recover her interests in people and things, but she no longer shows any signs of the previous symptoms which had made her a domestic virago and a social menace. Her husband is the greatest lithium enthusiast in East Kent, and I have no doubt that it saved the marriage.

I have also been studying the effect of the drug in a small group of four cases of manic–depressive personality. The diagnosis is not always easy to make, and there are often factors other than endogenous to complicate the picture, so I should prefer not to comment on any of these patients, except to mention a nineteen-year-old boy whose scholastic career was being constantly interrupted by manic mood-swings, who, under the influence of lithium over the last eighteen months, has been able to complete his school syllabus and to proceed to the London Polytechnic. Without treatment he would undoubtedly have had to leave school without taking the all-important examinations.

Finally, I have been experimenting with lithium on a group of seven patients with frequent recurrent depressions. There is little in the literature to suggest that depressive syndromes are improved by the drug and it is certainly not to be advocated during the acute depression episode, but I have been using it as a prophylactic against further depressions in these patients and have had very promising results in five of them, although admittedly follow-up has not so far been long enough to be very convincing. I submit to you the following two case histories.

A man of forty-seven first came under our care in 1948. There was no significant family history. He was regarded as having always been a rather ineffectual and inadequate person, subject to spells of depression. In the eight years following 1948 he attended out-patients from time to time and had a number of short courses of electroplexy, which usually produced a satisfactory if short-lived result. In 1956 his father and mother died within a month of each other and he became acutely depressed and showed some obsessional symptoms. He was admitted to hospital and recovered after five ECT, but he relapsed again in June and again in August, being re-admitted for electroplexy on each occasion. He continued, very reluctantly, to have ECT as an out-patient from time to time. His morale was getting very low and he regarded his medical advisers with well-merited suspicion and dread. In March 1958 he was with difficulty persuaded to take lithium regularly. After starting on 0.6 g t.d.s. he is now on a maintenance dose of 0.3 g b.d. and has remained symptom-free for the last eighteen months. His wife reports that during this period he has shown more self-confidence than ever before.

Another man, then aged forty-eight, came under our care in 1949. His father had suffered from recurrent depression and had finally committed suicide, and his mother had had a nervous illness of unknown nature lasting for two to three years in her middle life. In 1929 the patient was admitted to Netley Hospital after having attempted suicide by cutting his throat. He recovered from this depression and appears to have remained well until 1949 when he became depressed again, and was admitted to hospital. He received thirteen ECT and was discharged symptom-free, but he relapsed five months later and had to be re-admitted. Twelve further ECT produced a partial remission only and in July 1950 he underwent a prefrontal leucotomy. The depressive condition, however, continued to relapse and there were further hospital admissions in 1954, 1955 and twice in 1958. On all occasions he responded to electrotherapy fairly well but he was becoming increasingly averse to this form of treatment and would avoid consulting a doctor as long as possible. During his second admission in 1958 he was started on lithium carbonate 0.6 g t.d.s. He developed a severe tremor of the hands and a tic of the face, but the drug was persisted with at the lower dosage of 0.3 g t.d.s. and the tremors gradually subsided. He distrusted the drug intensely and stated he had lost all confidence in himself but he was persuaded to leave hospital and return to work. He has kept very well since and says that he feels better now than he has done for a long time. His present cheerful appearance at out-patients contrasts markedly with his former apprehensive and crestfallen demeanour.

To summarise, I have satisfied myself, if nobody else, that the drug is of real value in the treatment and particularly in the prevention of manic and hypomanic states, and that it has given promising results in the prevention of the more common condition of recurrent depression. I have little but the merest conjecture to offer about its mode of action. Apart from some electrocardiographic changes, which seem unimportant, and some electroencephalographic alterations, which I do not pretend to understand, its main action in the body seems to be on the balance of electrolytes. There is an increased excretion of cation (mainly sodium) and serum levels tend to fall. It has been recognised for some time that biochemical changes occur in periodic psychoses, and some recent work by Crammer has drawn attention to electrolyte changes in these patients, although whether these are primary or secondary is not definitely established. It is possible that lithium acts through this mechanism to modify the biochemical imbalance which may underlie periodic affective psychoses. Lithium belongs to the group of alkali metals. It stands at no. 3 in the atomic table, only hydrogen and helium having a smaller atomic weight. Thus it is the lightest of the solid elements and it is perhaps not surprising that it should in consequence possess certain modest magical qualities.

Index

Note: in this index, the names of individuals are quoted in the fullest form which appears anywhere in the text.